All in a Doctor's Day

A Collection of Short Medical Stories

by

Peter Sykes

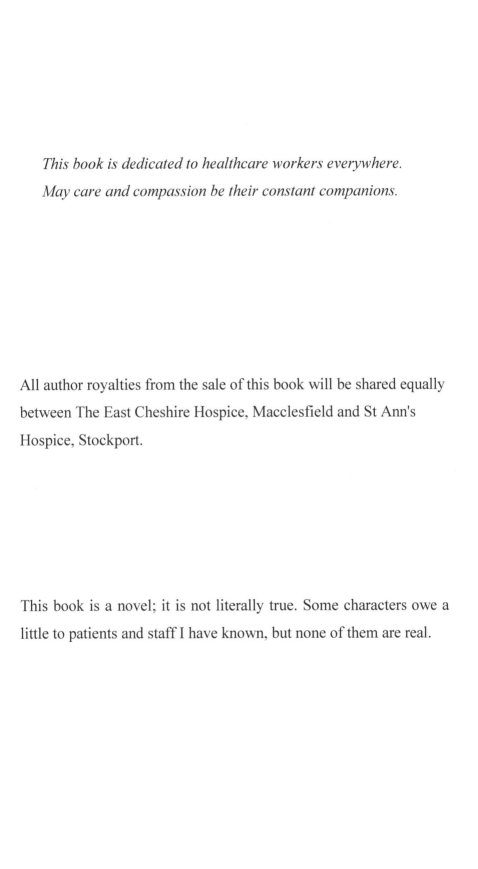

This book is dedicated to healthcare workers everywhere.
May care and compassion be their constant companions.

All author royalties from the sale of this book will be shared equally between The East Cheshire Hospice, Macclesfield and St Ann's Hospice, Stockport.

This book is a novel; it is not literally true. Some characters owe a little to patients and staff I have known, but none of them are real.

Acknowledgements

I wish to thank my wife Jane for her patience and for the numerous cups of tea (and the occasional glass of wine) that have sustained me whilst writing these stories.

Ideas for the stories have come from many different sources and in this regard I wish to acknowledge the contributions made by Ian Gibson, Geoff Leigh-Ford, Ricky Marcus, Graham Ostick, Bill Smith, Steve Spiro, Robert Sykes, Ken Tuson and Paul Willis.

I also offer my thanks to the many patients it has been my privilege to serve for giving me the inspiration to write this book.

By the same author

Peter's first novel **'The First Cut'** was published in 2011. It described Paul Lambert's medical misadventures as he was thrown, bewildered and unprepared, onto a busy surgical ward as a newly qualified doctor.

This was followed in 2013 by **'Behind the Screens'** which tells real-life tales at a time when care and compassion ruled supreme in British hospitals. Some of the stories are humorous, some sad, others poignant, but all are very 'human'. The novel also follows Paul's chequered love life and unveils some of the 'high jinks' that doctors get up to when off-duty.

'First Do No Harm' published in 2015, is set against the political disputes that beset the National Health Service between 1974 and 1976. Again the narrative is interspersed with numerous fascinating tales of the patients treated by Paul and his medical and nursing colleagues.

'Invisible Scars' was published in 2017. Paul, now training to become a surgeon, and his wife Nurse Kate, work alongside each other on a surgical unit. Strains in their relationship emerge. And when Kate's baby dies and Paul's inexperience costs lives, doubt and despair hang in the air and their marriage appears to be doomed.

However, in a dramatic turn of events, Paul saves the life of a critically ill patient and Kate is finally able to bid an emotional farewell to the child she has lost.

Preface

Peter Sykes has been steeped in medicine from the day he was born. His father was a doctor who consulted from the family home and his mother was a nurse, so it was perhaps no surprise when he too studied to be a doctor. Jane, his wife, is also medically qualified, and their marriage has been blessed with three sons, all of whom currently work for the NHS: as a physiotherapist, a general practitioner and as a clinical academic. Now retired, Peter has a wide breadth of experience having served as a hospital consultant, as medical director to an NHS Trust that provided hospital, community and mental health services and as a consultant to the Healthcare Commission.

This selection of short stories reflects his life time's experience of medical events. Some of the events related actually happened, some might have happened had certain situations developed differently and some are entirely fictional. They embrace a wide variety of healthcare personnel and situations, and every decade is represented from the 1960s to the present day. A few of the stories are tragic, others humorous and many have an unexpected twist in the tail.

Peter continues to publish new stories on his blog at www.medicaltales.org where you can Sign On/Subscribe and receive all future tales, free of charge, direct to your email in-box.

List of Chapters

Despair

Utterly dejected, I collapsed into the dilapidated armchair in the corner of the room, my head in my hands, tears in my eyes, my confidence shattered. I was distraught; my mood one of total wretchedness and despair. I was sweating and felt faint, my mouth was dry, and my hands trembled. It was four in the morning, and it was the events of those four hours, events for which I had been wholly responsible, that were the cause of my distress. What had happened had been a nightmare, an utter and complete disaster.

I had been the leader of the team, the one everyone respected, the one to whom they turned for guidance, the one supposed to be in control, and able to cope in difficult situations; but the night's events had shown me to have been a total failure. I was ashamed. I had let myself down, had let the team down and still lying on the operating table in the adjacent theatre, drained of his life-giving blood, was the man who paid the ultimate price for my incompetence.

The previous evening, William Wilson had been fit and well. He had enjoyed a lively game of bowls, followed by a drink and a chat with his pals in the pub. Now the nurses were washing the blood from his lifeless body in preparation for its short journey to the hospital morgue. Later, they would clean the operating table, scrub the floor, and sterilise the surgical instruments in preparation for the next day's list. By morning, the theatre would again be spotless, all evidence of the disaster that had unfolded in the night erased. If only they could wash away my shame, my pain, and my guilt as easily.

During my surgical training, I had grown accustomed to the occasional disappointment. There had been lows in my life before, times when patients had developed complications from treatments I had initiated, such things were inevitable for anyone who chose medicine as a career, but I had never experienced anything as terrible as this. If only the ground would open up and swallow me.

I glanced around the room, my eyes vaguely noting the jumble of discarded caps, masks, vests and pants left behind by the rest of the team as, one by one, they had drifted wearily to their beds, leaving me alone with my misery. Loyally, they had muttered words of sympathy, insisting that I should not blame myself; but their words brought no comfort. I did blame myself; who else was there to blame? My eye settled on the laundry-skip in the corner of the room.

A loose fold of a gown, heavily stained with blood, hung at an odd angle over the metal ring that formed its lip. A crimson pool was forming where blood was dripping onto the floor.

It brought to mind an image that had haunted me as a child. Whilst on a family holiday, I had seen hundreds of dead pheasants, their bloodied heads hanging limply, at grotesque angles over the side of a trailer, leaving a trail of blood on the rutted earth as they passed. The sight of their ruffled feathers and shattered bodies had sickened me. Walking alongside were half a dozen men, laughing and joking as they drank beer, their guns over the shoulders. Only a few hours before, we had fed the pheasants by hand as they roamed freely through our campsite. They had strutted proudly, bright-eyed, their heads held high, showing off the brilliant colours of their beautiful plumage: iridescent reds, brilliant greens, and blues. I suffered nightmares for weeks afterwards.

I looked again at the crumpled blood-stained gown. Poor Mr Wilson had died just as needlessly as those birds, and in my heart, I knew that I was responsible.

There was a quiet knock at the door and the theatre sister entered, a mug of tea in her hand.

'It's been a long night, Doctor,' she said, a sad, sympathetic smile on her face. 'Here, have a drink before you leave.'

I mumbled my thanks, head bowed, not trusting myself to look her in the eye.

'Look, you mustn't blame yourself. We must accept that from time to time, these things happen; not all operations are successful. If all your patients made a full recovery, you wouldn't be human; you'd be a miracle worker. Besides, when a major blood vessel bursts there's high mortality, you know that as well as I do. Had Mr Wilson not had surgery he would have died. You tried to save him; you did your best, no-one could ask for more.'

'And my best wasn't good enough, was it, Sister?'

Sister laid a hand on my shoulder. I wanted to shrug it off but didn't. 'Not this time maybe,' she said softly, 'but I've no doubt that others you operate on in the future will survive. Now, drink your tea and go to bed.'

Alone again, I took off my theatre greens, pulled on my shirt and pants, and looked in the mirror. A pale, unshaven, weary face looked back at me. I stared at it in disgust.

'Bloody idiot,' I muttered, cursing the ambition and misplaced ego that had reduced me to this state. 'What the hell are you doing trying to become a surgeon? You haven't the skill to be a success, nor the strength, the resilience to deal with the pain of failure.'

Then, turning away from the mirror, I collected my white coat and braced myself for the task that would compound my misery. I had to meet Mrs Wilson and tell her that her husband had not survived my surgery.

Thought for the day

Success has many fathers, while failure is an orphan.
Mid 20th Century Proverb

A Troubled Marriage

John, a General Practitioner in a suburban practice on the outskirts of York, set aside a couple of hours twice a week to undertake his clerical and administrative work. It was a chance for him to sit in his room, close the door, and work free of interruptions. He started by clearing the requests for repeat prescriptions. It didn't him take long and was an undemanding task. Then he reviewed the results of the blood tests and x-rays he'd requested on his patients. He had to decide who needed to be reviewed and who simply needed to be reassured their test results were normal.

He spent more time on the letters he'd received from hospital consultants about patients he had referred for a second opinion. They were always informative. Those who had simply been put on a surgical waiting list for a condition such as a rupture or varicose veins, he merely filed, but the ones that particularly interested him, were those where he had struggled to make sense of a patient's symptoms or was unsure of the best way to manage their condition. These were an opportunity to see what an expert in the appropriate field had made of the problem; an opportunity to learn.

Next, he moved on to the administrative matters that required his attention; directives from the Ministry of Health, and financial matters relating to the surgery. This was work that he knew was necessary but which he regarded as a chore. He was just thinking how much happier he would be, if medicine was simply a matter of looking after patients when there was a polite knock at the door.

'Come in,' he called.

It was Mary from the back office. 'We were just having a brew Doctor, and I thought you would like a cup of tea. And I've brought you a couple of those chocolate digestives too; I know they're your favourites.'

'Thanks, Mary, you're an angel.'

John lent back in his chair and started to reflect. He enjoyed his life as a General Practitioner and had been happy since he joined the High Melton Medical Centre. He liked the easy, friendly atmosphere in the surgery; he enjoyed a good relationship with the other doctors and, by and large, got on well with his patients. They represented a pleasant cross-section of the population. The practice covered an area on the edge of the city, including a large residential area, a small council estate, and one or two houses in the neighbouring countryside, occupied by the 'well-to-do', some of whom had joined the practice as private patients. Which reminded him, he'd better get back to these administrative matters, as he had arranged to see Jeanette Hopkins at Melton Manor on his way home. A frown creased his brow; she'd been worrying him; she didn't look well, and he found her symptoms difficult to assess. Maybe she was someone on whom he ought to be seeking a consultant's opinion.

John was met at the door by Mrs Hopkins' cleaner.

'Mrs Hopkins is upstairs in bed,' she said, 'and not for the first time,' she added, meaningfully. 'You can find your way, Doctor, can't you - up the stairs and the first door on the left? It's the big front bedroom with the bow window and the en-suite.'

John found Mrs Hopkins in bed, a sleeping mask over her eyes and with the curtains drawn. Forty-five years of age, she looked pale and tired.

'I'm sorry to trouble you like this, Doctor, but I feel tired all the time.'

Inwardly John groaned; they had lots of patients who complained of being 'Tired All The Time', – so many in fact that they referred to them as 'TATTS'. It was a modern epidemic; most of them had nothing wrong with them at all!

'And I have this awful headache as well,' Mrs Hopkins continued. 'It's been bad for three or four days now, and I don't seem to be able to shake it off. I couldn't possibly have come to the surgery to wait with the other patients.'

John took a quick history. The pain was situated just above the eyes and was present most of the time, but there was little to suggest its cause. Her temperature was normal, as was her blood pressure. There was nothing to suggest anything serious was amiss.

'It may be a bit of a viral infection,' he said, 'but stress can often be a factor. Are you under any pressure, or is there perhaps something that's particularly worrying you at the moment?'

'No, I don't think so; well nothing serious anyway. There was a bit of a 'to do' at the bridge club recently. Anne Tetley and I had a little disagreement when she made a false bid, and then tried to change it. But we called the adjudicator, and he said I was in the right. She's been a bit standoffish with me since.'

John started to gather his things together. 'Right, I'll give you something to ease your headache but I'm sure it will pass in a couple of days.'

'That's very kind of you, Doctor, I appreciate you visiting me. Will the tablets help my backache too?'

This remark caused John to make a few enquiries about her back pain, but again he found nothing amiss. Becoming increasingly certain that anxiety and stress were Mrs Hopkins basic problem, he decided to play amateur psychologist and began to probe a little deeper.

'You say you have no major worries, how are things at home?'

'No real problems, Doctor, well, no more than other couples, I guess.'

'And how are things between you and your husband?' John asked cautiously, aware that he was now moving into personal territory.

'Well, Doctor, I do get lonely. Arthur works in the city and has to commute to work. He's off at the crack of dawn each morning and he doesn't get home until late in the evening. As a result, I'm on my own a lot. And he's the president of the golf club too; that takes up a lot of his time at the weekend. So the truth is, I don't see a lot of him. But if it's the matrimonial side of things you're asking about Doctor, well, no - we don't often have relations. In fact, I can't remember the last time we had sex. At night, Arthur gives me a quick peck on the cheek, turns over, and is asleep in two minutes. Then I lie there, tossing and turning, listening to him grunting and snoring. And in bed at night, my legs are restless. I read something recently in the Daily Mail about restless legs, but apparently, there's not a lot you can do about them. With one thing and another, I find it difficult to get any sleep at all, and then, of course, I'm tired when I wake up in the morning. In fact, Doctor, I was wondering if you could help me with some sleeping pills.'

John was becoming ever more certain, that all his patient's troubles were due to stress, and a burned-out marriage.

'Have you thought of taking a holiday, having a break?'

'It's strange that you should say that, Doctor. Arthur's dad and his new wife have asked us to go with them to Cyprus, but I really don't think I could go.'

'It sounds as if it could be a good way of getting to know her, and the sunshine and fresh air would do you good,' John commented.

'Oh, I get along with her all right, but the problem is they're planning to take her son along as well...,' she hesitated before going on, '....well, I just don't think it would work.'

'And this young man, what is his name?'

'He's called James.'

'And don't you get on with him?'

Mrs Hopkins lips melted into a warm smile. 'I get on with him very well. He's lovely, quite the opposite of Arthur. He's lively, quick-witted, delightful company – and so good looking. I'd like to see much more of him, but that would be a bit awkward.'

'Do you see him often?'

'Yes, I try to see him whenever Arthur is away.'

John was sure he was now getting to the root of Mrs Hopkins' problems. She had a guilty secret – she was in love. He wondered how far her romance had progressed, and whether her husband had any suspicions.

'And you're fond of him?'

Mrs Hopkins whole attitude changed. She came to life, her eyes sparkled, a smile lit up her face. 'Yes, I adore him. Whenever I'm with him, I want to hold him in my arms, hug him, and feel close to him. He makes me so happy; it makes me realise what I've been missing all these years.'

'And does he love you in return?'

'Oh yes, definitely. He's so sweet. Only the other day, he said he wanted to marry me.'

John wondered if she realised that if, or perhaps when, her husband discovered her infidelity, her life would become even more stressful.

'Look,' he said, 'I'm sure it's very flattering for a lady of your age to have a sexy young man attracted to you, but you need to think very carefully before you take things too far. There's your marriage to think about, your home, your whole lifestyle.'

'Oh, Doctor, you've got it all wrong. James is only six years old and I love him so very much. If only it would have been possible for me to have a child of my own.'

John saw the tears well up in her eyes, and realised he had finally stumbled on the cause of his patient's unhappiness. He reached out and took her hand.

The Telephonist's Tale

'Hello; you're through to the Middleton Hospital, good morning.' If Sarah had said that once, she had said it ten thousand times. She had been the senior telephonist at the hospital for many years. It was a job she loved, and she prided herself on her efficiency.

'Get me Davies, will you,' instructed the caller.

Surprised by the caller's tone, Sarah paused before replying.

'We have a couple of gentlemen in the hospital called Davies, which Mr Davies do you wish to contact?'

'Davies on the medical unit.'

'Oh you mean, Doctor Davies,' Sarah replied, emphasising the word Doctor. She held the hospital's senior physician in high regard.

'Yes, Dr Davies, and be quick about it.'

The caller's tone upset Sarah. 'May I enquire who's calling, please?'

'My name's irrelevant. Now hurry, will you? I've not got all day!'

It was Tuesday morning, and Sarah knew that Dr Chris Davies would be seeing patients in the Out-Patient Department and wouldn't wish to be interrupted unnecessarily.

'Perhaps you could tell me the nature of your call?'

'No, I can't; damn you. It's confidential. Just put me through!'

Sarah was not accustomed to being spoken to in this fashion but remained professional. 'Please hold the line, and I'll see if he is available.'

She put the caller on hold, and then rang the clinic where Dr Davies took the call. The minute the line was cleared, she rang the clinic again where the consultant picked up the phone.

'Hello, Dr Davies,' she said, 'this is Sarah from the switchboard.'

The consultant knew her well. She was a longstanding colleague in the hospital and had been a patient of his as well.

'Hi Sarah, what can I do for you?'

'I wonder if you would tell me whom it was that called you a moment or two ago.'

Dr Davies frowned; it was an unusual request.

'Why do you want to know Sarah?'

'Really to let you know that he's the rudest man I've ever had to deal with, in all the years I've worked here.'

'Oh dear, Sarah. I'm sorry if he upset you. His name is David Bartram-Smythe. He's an applicant for the vacant consultant job we have in the Medical Department.'

'Would that be the Dr Bartram-Smythe who worked here as a junior doctor a couple of years ago?'

'Yes it would; do you remember him?'

'I certainly do, and at the risk of speaking out of turn, may I say I hope he won't be appointed.'

So do I, Dr Davies thought, though he held his words in check. 'Thank you, Sarah,' he said, 'that's useful feedback. I'll bear it in mind.'

Later that week, Chris Davies and his consultant colleagues, amongst them Jim O'Connor and Frank Taylor, met to discuss the forthcoming appointment. Chris opened the meeting by relaying his conversation with Sarah. This surprised no-one. They all remembered Dr David Bartram-Smythe, or DBS as he was always called. Though academically brilliant, his time working at the Middleton had been a disaster. His superior demeanour, and his rude and dismissive attitude towards those he considered inferior had caused endless trouble. Several times he had been advised as to his behaviour, but it had made little difference. Everyone had been pleased when he left for a post at a prestigious London teaching hospital.

'Our problem,' Jim remarked 'is that on paper, he's a very strong candidate. He has an excellent CV. He has a higher degree, he's done some important research, and his references have been written by some high-flying people, a couple of professors amongst them.'

'That may be true,' Frank replied, 'but when he was here before, he caused endless trouble with his arrogance, his 'holier-than-thou' attitude and his rudeness to the nurses. If you remember, there were disputes about the duty roster and arguments about holidays. Worst still, he upset patients on numerous occasions. I don't want him to return, especially as a permanent member of staff.'

'I agree,' Jim said. 'This has always been a good hospital in which to work. It's a friendly place, with a pleasant atmosphere. Most of the staff are local, they're loyal, and everyone gets on well together. We've worked hard to build that reputation, we mustn't risk destroying it.'

'Then we must make sure he's not appointed,' Chris said. 'I'll find out who will be on the interview panel, and see what I can do.'

Dr Davies' enquiries, however, left him more pessimistic than ever. There were to be seven members on the interviewing panel; a professor of medicine from London, representatives from the University and the Royal College, two lay members, one of them acting as chairman, and only two, Chris himself and the hospital's chief executive, from the Middleton. Chris could envisage exactly what would happen. Bartram-Smythe would turn on the charm and sweet-talk the lay members, and then impress the academics with his research achievements. When it came to deciding on the appointment, they would lose the argument by five votes to two. At a stroke, the happy, sociable atmosphere that existed in the hospital, and particularly on the medical wards, would be destroyed. Last time this troublemaker had worked with them, he had been on a twelve-month contract. That had been bad enough; now he would become a permanent member of staff.

Meanwhile, the matter was widely debated on the hospital's grapevine, and it became obvious that the possibility of DBS returning was causing considerable disquiet. One of the ward sisters even said that he upset patients so much that she would leave if she had to work with him again.

Three candidates had been selected for an interview; DBS and two others, either of whom Dr Davies would have welcomed with open arms. But as the date of the appointment approached, he had a deep sense of foreboding. At the interview, he could stress to the other members of the panel, the need to maintain the pleasant atmosphere and harmony that existed within the hospital, but he knew that such a soft argument would count for naught with the majority of the panel.

The big day arrived, and as was usual, the candidates were to be interviewed in alphabetical order. DBS would be seen second.

The first candidate was called into the room. The interview lasted some 40 minutes, but at its conclusion, there was no sign of Dr Bartram-Smythe.

'Obviously, he isn't interested in the job.' Chris Davies remarked, clearly hoping that his application could be dismissed, 'I suggest that we proceed without him.'

But the chairman was having none of it. 'He's probably just been delayed by the traffic,' he said. 'We'll see the third candidate next, and interview him later.'

When the third candidate had also been interviewed, and DBS still hadn't arrived, Dr Davies, now beginning to feel slightly more optimistic, again suggested that his application be discounted. The chairman, however, asked that he be contacted, to determine his whereabouts. It was his wife who answered the phone.

'Oh dear,' she said, 'didn't he let you know. He decided to withdraw his application. There's a vacancy in Southampton that he would prefer.'

To Dr Davies' great relief, the committee appointed the stronger of the two remaining candidates. He left the room with a huge smile on his face and immediately rang the switchboard, to contact his colleagues to tell them the good news. It happened to be Sarah, who was on duty.

'Are the interviews over?' she asked eagerly. 'Did that dreadful man turn up?'

'No, as it happened, he didn't. But what made you ask that? Did you think that he might not attend?'

'I just thought he might be put off by the rumours that are circulating about the Middleton being downgraded to a cottage hospital; you know, losing its maternity, paediatric and emergency departments, and so on.'

'But that's nonsense. There aren't any such rumours. It's the very opposite, in fact. We've been selected for development. Ten million is coming our way for a new pathology lab and x-ray department.'

'Oh dear,' Sarah said innocently, 'I must have misled the poor man. I bumped into him when he came to look round the hospital a couple of weeks ago. For some reason, he thought I was the hospital's general manager. I'm very sorry, Dr Davies; I'll make sure those rumours about becoming a cottage hospital go no further.'

The Visiting Angel

When patients are grateful for the care they receive, be it in hospital, in the GP's surgery, or at home, they frequently express their gratitude by offering small gifts to the doctors and nurses. The doctors are *'marvellous'*, and may be given a bottle of wine or whisky, the nurses are *'angels'*, and tend to receive chocolates or biscuits. Such praise and recognition are great motivating factors. But what of all the other equally essential members of the team: the clerical staff, the paramedics, porters, cooks, cleaners, management, and maintenance staff, without whose contributions the front-line staff couldn't operate? Their contributions are just as important, but all too often, their role in the patient's care is overlooked. I hope this little story helps to redress the balance.

***

As soon as the doctor entered the room, I could tell that something was wrong; it was the expression on his face, the sadness in his eyes. He had been kind, he'd broken the news to me as gently as he could, but I was devastated. Afterwards, the nurse had sat with me for a long time, brought me a cup of tea, and offered comfort. Whilst she had been with me, I had been brave, I'd held back my tears but now, alone in my room, they flowed freely.

I slipped out of bed and gazed into the cot. There he was, my Joe, my first-born baby son, just two weeks old. He was fast asleep, so beautiful, so peaceful, so unaware. Gently, I picked him up and, holding him in my arms, went back to bed. He stirred, and for a moment, his eyes opened, but almost immediately, he went back to sleep.

I held him, tight to my chest, feeling a mother's need to protect him from the world into which he had been born and, as I rocking him gently from side to side, murmuring sweet nothings into his ear, I reflected on how dramatically my life had changed. A year ago, I hadn't had a care in the world. I held a steady job, Craig had just moved in with me; we were happy, healthy, and everything looked rosy. My Mum had never liked Craig, said that she didn't trust him, and how right she had been. He'd turned out to be a two-timing bastard. I was devastated when I found out, but my Mum had helped me through, well mothers always do, don't they? At the time, I didn't realise I was pregnant – that came as a real shock. Inevitably, well-meaning friends offered their advice on what I should do, but it was Mum again who helped me make the right decision.

'I was a single mum,' she had said, 'you wouldn't be here if I'd had an abortion, would you?'

Well, that decided me, but at the time, I really hadn't appreciated just how much my life would change.

I was still lying in bed feeling sorry for myself, rocking baby Joe in my arms, when there was a knock on the door. I shouted 'come in', presuming it would be one of the nurses, or possibly the domestic coming to collect the remains of my lunch. The door opened slowly, and a little old man hobbled in, a walking stick in one hand. He must have been in his sixties, or possibly even older. He had unfashionably long, grey hair and a straggling beard, but it was his face that I particularly noticed. It was the face of a genial grandfather, soft features, bright eyes, and skin creases that seemed to smile at you. He wore a volunteer's badge on his lapel.

'I just popped in to see if you had time for a chat,' he said. He spoke with a soft Scottish accent but had a slight speech impediment which meant having to listen carefully to catch his words.

Quite why I said 'Yes', I truly don't know. Maybe I felt sorry for him because he was disabled, maybe I would have reproached myself for being unsociable had I sent him away, maybe it was something about the sparkle in his eyes, but I'm so glad now that I said 'Yes'.

He introduced himself as John, drew up a chair at the side of my bed, sat down, and we got talking. I can't recall now how the conversation started; maybe it was about the weather or the hospital food, but he avoided any personal matters. He had an easy, cheerful manner, a good sense of humour, and an uplifting manner; all in all, he was pleasant company. As we spoke, I noticed his hand was clenched tightly, and I realised that he must have the same condition as my baby, Joe. Since we had something in common, I plucked up courage and asked him if he'd had the trouble with his hand ever since he was a baby.

'Yes,' he said, 'I'm spastic, well, that's what I was told when I was a kid. It affects my left side; my leg as well as my arm, and I'm guessing you will have noticed my words aren't as clear as I'd like them to be.'

There was no hint of self-pity in his voice and no change in the gentle smile on his lips.

'I gather it's called cerebral palsy now,' I said, 'I've just been told that my little boy has it.'

'Ah, is that so?' he said and began to talk about his life. It became apparent that he had been far more severely affected than my Joe. He told me that for 40 years, he had worked in the office of a large insurance firm. He'd enjoyed life there, had played for the office darts team, and made lifelong friends.

'I didn't take any more time off work than any of my workmates,' he said proudly.

He played bowls and had fulfilled two major ambitions; to have a pint of beer in every pub in his home town and to attend a football match at every league club in the country. He had a collection of football programmes to prove it!

He'd never married and had been living on his own for 12 years since his mother died. As he spoke, it literally brought a tear to my eye. John was obviously at the more severe end of hemiplegia, my Joe being very much milder in comparison, but there he was, as happy as anything, telling me how wonderful his life had been.

As John left, he probably didn't know that hearing his story had changed my attitude to my baby's condition. I'd felt so low when the doctors explained Joe's problems to me, but John had shown me there was no reason why he shouldn't lead a full, happy, and purposeful life.

I am so grateful for that knock at the door, and so pleased I didn't turn John away. So thank you for dropping by, John. You're an angel.

Thought for the day

Imperfect people can make the world a better place.
Ken Follett 1949.......

A memorable night

There was an unmarked door in the heart of the Casualty Department. It opened into a tiny room with bare, plastered walls. The room had no windows, being lit by a single, unshaded bulb set into the low ceiling. There was scarcely enough space for the bed. Apart from a small bedside locker, there was no other furniture; no chair, no drawers, not even a hook on the door on which to hang a coat. The moment I entered, I started to sweat, it was hot, airless and oppressive. A four-inch, cast-iron central heating pipe, devoid of any lagging, ran the length of the room, acting as an oversized radiator. I touched it, then snatched my fingers away, afraid of being burned. The room was so claustrophobic; I doubted I should get a wink of sleep, even without the responsibility that had been heaped on my shoulders.

I was 23 years old, had been qualified for just two weeks, and I was to be the only doctor in the Department for the rest of the night. It was 2 am, and I was to be 'first on-call' for the next seven hours. I was ill-equipped for the job, and wondered whether I would cope.

In the sixties and seventies, it was common practice for the responsibility for treating patients with medical emergencies to be placed on the shoulders of the most junior and least-experienced doctors in the hospital who, more often than not, were also the most exhausted. It was an arrangement that wasn't safe, either for the doctors or the patients. These days, Accident and Emergency Departments all have permanent staff led by highly-trained consultants. The doctors come on duty as a team, work their eight or ten-hour shifts, and then go off duty. They don't do a full day's work on the wards and then do a solo night shift in Casualty, before working for a further day back on the ward as we did. Mind you, in days gone by, far fewer patients attended Casualty than they do today, especially in the early hours of the morning.

Others who had undertaken this duty before me had offered reassurance. The Nursing Sisters, they said, were senior and very experienced. They would help, guide, and mother me and, hopefully, see me through. And I knew that more senior doctors could be called from the main hospital if necessary, but nevertheless, the prospect of being in charge was daunting.

Since the waiting room was now empty, I retired to the cubbyhole that was to be my bedroom for the night. I stripped to my underpants and lay on top of the sheets hoping to find sleep, but within 15 minutes, I was called to attend to a new arrival. Fortunately, it proved to be no more than a sprained wrist. I organised a bandage and some pain relief, returned to my room and, hot and stuffy though it was, drifted into a heavy sleep.

It must have been about three in the morning when the phone rang. It felt as though I hadn't been asleep for more than two or three minutes, although the clock insisted that an hour had passed since I'd retired. The patient was a lad of 19 years who was clearly drunk. He was unable to give a coherent account of himself, but his mates said he'd fallen down some steps on his way home from one of the nightclubs in the city centre.

Inexperienced though I was, it was obvious from the gross deformity that his ankle was broken. The next step was an x-ray to determine the nature and extent of his fracture. This meant a phone call to the duty radiographer, who I presumed would be tucked up in bed, probably in the Nurses' Home. Nurses and female radiographers were locked up at night at a safe distance from the doctors' residency!

Confident that I was following correct procedure, I rang her and apologised for disturbing her. I explained about the lad with the ankle injury and invited her (with an appropriate 'please' and 'thank you' as becomes a newly qualified doctor) to confirm my diagnosis, so that future treatment could be planned. I remembered one of the senior physicians advising that you should never *'order'* an x-ray or a blood test; you should always *'request'* one.

A long pause followed, so long, in fact, I thought that in her sleepy state, she hadn't understood what I'd said.

I was just about to repeat my request when she spoke. Her aggressive tone alarmed me.

'What the bloody hell do you expect me to do about it at this time of the night?'

'Well, since it's clearly fractured, I thought it might be appropriate to get it x-rayed,' I said, recovering sufficiently to add a trace of sarcasm to my voice.

'And what on earth would be the point of that?' she snapped back. 'Will you be able to anaesthetise him whilst he is drunk? Do you suppose that the surgeons are going to reduce the fracture in the middle of the night? Don't they teach you anything at Medical School these days? For God's sake; immobilise it, relieve his pain, and send him to the x-ray department in the morning.'

With a bang, the telephone receiver went down.

My first response was to feel angry. I wasn't responsible for the lad's broken ankle. I'd been perfectly polite to her, what right did she have to be so rude to me?

However, on reflection, and having discussed the situation with the nursing sister in charge of the department, I had to admit that she was right. Nothing would be gained from x-raying him at three in the morning. It made me realise that whilst I had a great deal of medical knowledge (well, at least sufficient to pass the final medical school exam!) my training had left me inadequately prepared for the practicalities of medical life. I hadn't been taught how healthcare is actually delivered in practice; the emphasis on learning facts had come at the expense of acquiring practical skills.

Back I went to my cubby hole and again drifted off to sleep.

I was awakened by a knock on the door, and one of the nurses walked in.

'Wakey-wakey,' she said cheerfully, sounding like Billy Cotton at the beginning of his 'Big Band Show'.

'It's seven-thirty in the morning, time to rise and shine.'

She had sparkling blue eyes and a generous smiling mouth, set in a full round face, framed with curly dark hair. It was, however, her hourglass figure that was most striking, acting as a magnet to my gaze. Moll Flanders in a nurse's uniform. With the top three buttons of her dress undone, she revealed far more of her generous cleavage than Matron's regulations on nurses' uniforms allowed. I felt my face flush and my senses quicken.

'I've brought you a cup of tea, Rob,' she said, using my Christian name in a further breach of Matron's rules, although we'd never met before.

The bedside locker was on the far side of the bed and the obvious thing was to walk around the foot of the bed and place the tea on the locker. This however, was not her way of doing things. Instead, she leant across the bed, her cleavage a few inches from my face. Despite the weariness I felt from my lack of sleep, the view of her breasts and the smell of her perfume proved intoxicating, indeed stimulating. Having placed the drink on the locker, she feigned to slip and steadied herself with a hand on my bare shoulder, her face directly in front of me, her lips only a couple of inches from mine. For one dreadful moment, I thought she was going to throw her arms around me and kiss me.

'We like to look after the doctors here,' she said, her voice husky and suggestive, 'especially the good-looking ones.'

Others, I'm sure, would have relished the situation, responded with some clever remark or witticism but I was embarrassed and tongue-tied. Conscious that I was dressed only in my underpants, I quickly drew the sheet up under my chin.

'Don't be shy, Rob,' she said, 'I'm a nurse; I've seen it all before.'

She sat down on the bed, just the sheet separating her shapely knee from my thigh. I could feel its warmth through the thin material.

'The night staff is going off duty now, but I've got a quickie for you.' Again, there was the suggestive voice and smile. I must have looked alarmed for she added, 'Don't worry; I'm not going to eat you. Mind you, you do look rather tasty.'

She put her finger on my nose and then very slowly traced a path downwards across my lips, caressing each in turn. The finger lingered on my chin and then seductively stroked my neck and upper chest until its descent was arrested by the sheet that I was holding tightly across my body. Her eyes had been following the course of her finger, but now they found mine; her smile teasing and provocative.

'Never mind,' she said wickedly, 'there's always next time.'

She retreated a foot or so, and I began to feel less vulnerable. Fortunately, she then became more business-like and told me of the patients who had attended the department whilst I'd been asleep.

'There's a man with a cut on his knee in cubicle one. We've sewn it up, and he's agreed to stay to let you see him. There are also three sets of notes for you to sign.'

'What are they?' I asked, puzzled.

'Patients we've seen while you've been asleep. We didn't want to wake you, so we've sorted them out. We just need you to sign the cards before you leave.'

'But how can I sign the records if I haven't seen the patients?'

'Oh, you are the innocent one, aren't you?' she said. 'We'll have to do something about that. Well, most doctors just sign the notes as if they have seen the patients. The alternative is for you to say that we treated them, but that they didn't wait to be seen by you.'

'But that's not quite true either, is it?' I replied.

The playful voice returned. 'You take things too seriously, Rob; I can see that I shall have to give you some personal tuition, show you how to relax and have a good time. Strictly speaking, it isn't true, but doing it this way saves you getting up every twenty minutes to see the patients who dribble in through the night. You should be grateful; we've given you a couple of hours of sleep. Anyway, I'll leave the cards out, and you can decide what you want to do with them. I must dash.'

Suddenly, the voice became suggestive again. 'It's been nice meeting you, Rob.' She fingered the top of the sheet that separated us. 'I hope to see much more of you very soon.'

She bent forward and gave me a quick kiss on the forehead. Again, there was an intoxicating mix of cleavage and perfume. She moved to leave, but by the door she turned, a twinkle in her eye and a smile on her lips.

'By the way, I'm moving to your ward next week. I'll see you there.'

I drank the cup of tea in bed wondering what I should do about the patients whom the nurses had seen and discharged during the night. Then I got dressed,

I reviewed the patient whose knee they had stitched, wrote in his medical record, and discharged him. I signed the other three cards, having recorded that the patients hadn't waited to be seen. I wasn't happy about doing this, but at least there was an element of truth in it. Hopefully there would be no comeback.

Whilst writing up the case notes, I heard the sound of activity and, leaving the office, found two of the surgical cubicles occupied. The receptionist had taken up her position for the new day and a new team of nurses, all bright and cheerful, had come on duty. I felt the stubble on my chin and then put a hand to my armpit; there was an unmistakable smell of body odour.

Sister took me to one side, and her words were most welcome. 'Although you're officially on duty until nine,' she said, 'I suggest you go to the residency and freshen up. If anything urgent turns up, we'll bleep you. Any other cases can wait and be seen by the Casualty officers when they come on duty at eight thirty.'

I walked slowly back to the residency, feeling hungry, tired, and light-headed. The nursing staff who had shared the night work with me had been off-duty the day before, were off duty again now, and had enjoyed a meal break during the night, whereas I'd worked all day yesterday, through the night, and now, with my head still throbbing gently from the heat in the bedroom, faced another full day's work.

Back in the residency, I freshened up with a long, hot shower, and then went for breakfast. The other house officers, particularly those who had yet to work the graveyard shift in Casualty were keen to know how I'd fared. I related the experience of my early morning cup of tea.

'That will be Sue Weston,' someone said. 'She's got quite a reputation. If she's coming to your ward, you'd better watch your step.'

I felt much better when breakfast was over. Somehow bacon, eggs, toast, marmalade, and a large mug of coffee established a baseline for the day, and the slight disorientation I'd felt when leaving the Casualty department disappeared. I also felt a sense of satisfaction. I had come through my first night as a Casualty officer. It had been tough – but I had survived.

Thought for the Day

'Do you want to speak to the Doctor in Charge or to the nurse who really knows what's going on?'

Author unknown

An interesting Heart Murmur

I am certain that many folk reading this, certainly the older ones amongst you, will remember a book written by Dr Richard Gordon entitled 'Doctor in the House'. He worked for a time as an anaesthetist at St Bartholomew's Hospital in London where he had been a medical student.

'Doctor in the House' was adapted into a very popular film in which Dirk Bogarde played the role of Simon Sparrow, a medical student. Perhaps the film's most memorable scene featured a group of students around a patient's bed being interrogated by the hospital's fearsome senior consultant, Sir Lancelot Spratt, played by James Robertson Justice.

The patient is being prepared for surgery, but has a blood clotting problem.

'What's the bleeding time?' Sir Lancelot roars at the group.

Poor Simon looks at his watch. 'Ten-thirty, sir,' he replies.

The following story has certain similarities, and is similarly embarrassing for the poor medical student concerned.

***

A group of five or six medical students were crowded around a hospital bed during the ward round of a senior and irascible consultant cardiologist. Also around the bed were the ward sister, and some of her junior nurses. One of the young students, to save his blushes I shall call him Tony Smithson, was asked to listen to the heart of the patient, and then describe to the group the murmur that he heard.

Tony was a quiet introspective young man, not one who felt comfortable in the limelight. Although a bright and diligent student, he was usually to be found at the back of the group trying to avoid being noticed. Nervously he took his stethoscope from the pocket of his white coat, and approached the patient. Politely, he asked if the patient would mind having his chest examined.

'Of course he doesn't mind,' the consultant snapped. 'He's come into hospital to be examined and treated hasn't he?'

'Er...yes, Sir... of course, he has, Sir,' Tony responded, his nerves beginning to get the better of him.

He opened the top button of the patient's pyjama jacket and applied the stethoscope to his chest.

'No, not like that! If you're going to listen to his chest, for Heaven's sake do the job properly. Take his pyjama top off completely.'

Tentatively, Tony placed a hand on the patient's chest to locate the apex beat as he had been instructed in a previous teaching session.

'My, your hands are cold,' the patient said.

'Sorry,' Tony replied, his pulse rising as he became increasingly stressed.

The consultant then added to his discomfort. 'I didn't say feel, I said listen.'

Becoming ever more anxious, Poor Tony became flustered. He listened to the patient's heart and, to his credit, despite the pressure he was under he was able, not only to hear the murmur, but to identify what it was. Furthermore, he knew the condition that caused it. The correct term was an '*ejection* murmur', but unfortunately after a moment's hesitation, the words that Tony uttered were an '*ejaculation* murmur'.

The other medical students thought this was hilarious, as did the nurses who fell about in fits of giggles.

He was teased about the episode unmercifully for weeks afterwards, especially as the consultant immediately asked, 'Whatever were you thinking about, Smithson?'

'Well, I er, Sir, I really should have said, er,' Tony began but before he could complete the sentence, the consultant added to his misery.

'Perhaps I should have asked *who* were you thinking about? Was it one of these pretty young nurses perhaps?' he asked.

Though everyone laughed, and thought the exchange had been hilarious, one of the nurses felt an immediate surge of sympathy for Tony. She had a motherly desire to hug and console him. Her name was Kate, but she had to wait three months, then take the initiative by asking him for a date, before her wish came true.

Anno Domini

As a young man, I often heard old folks remark, usually with a sad smile and a knowing shake of the head, '*Growing old is no fun, you know*'. At the time, I didn't take much notice but I'm now beginning to understand what they meant. I'm discovering that Old Father Time creeps up on you insidiously.

I was in my forties when I started to use reading glasses but found them to be a nuisance. When I was working in the surgery they were on, then off, then on again, as I alternated between reading the notes and focussing on my patient. Finding the situation unsatisfactory, I invested in some bifocals, but these proved to be a waste of money. It didn't matter whether I used the upper or the lower lens, the computer screen remained out of focus. In desperation, I bought some varifocal glasses which were more expensive still. They took a bit of getting used to, but proved to be a good investment and I now wear them all the time.

In my fifties, I became deaf in my left ear. For several years, a sense of misplaced pride caused me to shun a hearing aid but, eventually, tired of being told I was shouting, I had to accept that I needed it. It brought a dramatic improvement, the only downside being a greater awareness of the driving instructions coming from a certain lady sitting in the front passenger seat of the car. '*Left, left*', she would say, indicating wildly with her right hand. Yet more expense. I had to invest in a 'Satnav' to solve that problem.

In my sixties, I needed a hearing aid in the other ear. It was either that or divorce as my wife and I regularly came to blows over the volume control on the television. Why the BBC can't persuade their announcers to speak a little louder, and the actors in television dramas to enunciate their words more clearly, I shall never know. Again I resisted, but in the end I acquiesced, it was worth it for the domestic harmony that returned to our living room each evening. This brings me to another grouse. Why do folk seem to find deafness so amusing? Why don't they regard it with sympathy, as a medical affliction?

I'm now in my seventies, and though I'm pleased to report I still have my own teeth, I'm developing arthritis in a couple of joints; I guess a walking stick may soon be added to my list of medical aids. Despite being otherwise healthy, active and, I believe, still of sound mind, I'm beginning to wonder what's next: a walking frame, an in-dwelling catheter? I'm certainly realising what those old folk meant when they used to say *'enjoy yourself whilst you're young. There's nothing to commend old age.'*

The present problem is that my wife says I'm becoming doolally. I don't honestly believe that I am, though I'm prepared to admit I may not be very good at remembering names. I prefer to believe that I'm merely selective in what I choose to remember. If Jane, that's my lady wife, tells me that a distant cousin of hers has three children, well, that's fine, I'll try to remember it. But if she goes on to give me their names, ages, then tells me which one has passed grade four on the piano, and the names of their pets, I'm afraid those facts don't register in my memory bank. It's not that I deliberately ignore what I've been told, but my brain seems to decide that this information is surplus to requirements. If it's not likely to be relevant, my brain seems to say, *why bother to remember it?*

Recently though, I must admit that I've forgotten a couple of things I really ought to have remembered. There was that birthday card I was supposed to post to one of my wife's relatives, (no – not to the distant cousin who has three, or was it four children, one of whom played the guitar, or was it the flute). And there were the Euros I forgot to buy for our next holiday, and, unfortunately, our wedding anniversary – now that really did get me into trouble! There really was no excuse for overlooking it because, when I missed our anniversary last year, I made a forward planning note in my diary which I'd actually read a few days before the big day this year. Unfortunately, I then forgot to do anything about it!

Now I seem to be in trouble most of the time. If I'm busy in the garden, and a few moments late picking up the grandchildren from school; I'm a 'scatterbrain'. I'm 'empty-headed' if I forget to put out the rubbish, or come home without the most important item on the weekly shopping list.

Recently though, I saw my chance to turn the tables. It was Jane's turn to be forgetful. She'd promised to arrange for some flowers to be sent to a friend in hospital, and forgot to do it. *Great*, I thought, *now my chance to get even.*

I didn't say anything at the time, but made a mental note, that the next time she accused me of being forgetful, I would remind her of the flowers that didn't get sent.

I didn't have long to wait. Within a week, we ran out of milk and yes, - you've guessed it - it had been my job to call at the corner shop to buy some. I'd forgotten it, and was being reprimanded. *Now,* I thought, *an opportunity to get my own back, I'll remind her that I'm not the only one who's absent-minded.*

But dammit, I realised that I'd completely forgotten what it was that she had forgotten, that I had been so desperate to remember!

Thought for the day

> *To my deafness I'm accustomed,*
> *To my dentures I'm resigned,*
> *I can manage my bifocals,*
> *But how I miss my mind.*
>   Lord Home 1903 - 1995

A muddy night in Manchester

It was one of the wettest, windiest Novembers that Lancashire had ever known, and heaven knows, over the years, there have been plenty of them. Rainfall records had been broken, rivers had overflowed their banks, houses had been flooded and trees blown asunder. Bonfire night had been a washout, numerous football matches postponed due to waterlogged pitches, and root vegetables were rotting in the ground. It made me wonder if I'd done the right thing when leaving my post in Kent and moving to the North West. Mind you, had I not done that, I wouldn't have met Harry nor had my two lovely children.

As was my usual routine when doing night duty, I'd spent the morning in bed and got up in time to greet the children as they returned from school. They were both soaked; it had been raining all day. Why kids today go out in a morning without coats, I shall never understand. I know school cloakrooms are a thing of the past but surely they should have the sense to put a foldaway mac in their bags before they leave home in the morning? I'd spent the next hour drying their wet clothes and cheering them up with drinks of hot chocolate.

Fortunately, Harry came home early, so after giving them their tea, I was able to splash my way through the wind, rain and puddles, and get to work. I've always worked as a carer either in residential homes or in the community, so working in the hospital was a new experience for me. Somewhat to my surprise, I found myself enjoying it, and working night shifts had not been as disruptive as I thought it might have been.

At the hospital I rarely knew in advance to which department I would be allocated. I was sent wherever they were short staffed, but I didn't really mind this uncertainty, it was all good experience, and the staff were always pleased when I turned up, and usually were pleasant people with whom to work.

On this particular night, I was told to report to the Accident and Emergency Department. I cannot deny that I was apprehensive, as previously I'd always been sent to one of the long-stay wards where my previous experience was relevant. A & E was quite an eye opener. It was incredibly busy, and my heart leapt every time I heard the siren of an ambulance as they brought yet another patient to the hospital. Most of the patients genuinely seemed to be in need of urgent treatment but quite a number of those who were sitting waiting to be seen, appeared to have little the matter with them. I'm not a doctor or qualified nurse, of course, but it seemed to me that they could have waited and gone to see their GP in the morning, always supposing, of course, that their doctor had appointments available for them.

At first, Sister asked me to clean and tidy the cubicles after patients had vacated them. Later, I made drinks for the staff and some sandwiches for a couple of the patients. Then Sister called me over and said she had a special job for me.

'I'd like you to wash this young man for me, and then sit with him awhile,' she said. 'We think he's called Sean, but we're not absolutely certain about that.'

'What's the matter with him?' I asked.

'Well, the truth is we're not quite sure. He's obviously had far too much to drink and the paramedics say he's been involved in a road accident, though it seems he was the passenger and not the driver. He's probably got some drugs on board as well as the alcohol, though quite what sort of cocktail we don't yet know. But he's obviously high on something!'

The young man, lying on a trolley in a cubicle, was a sorry sight. He was cold, wet, and shivering. He appeared to be confused, looking around as if he couldn't understand quite where he was, and mumbling incoherently under his breath, which reeked of alcohol. He had a bruise on his forehead, vomit down his shirt, and the smell suggested he had soiled his trousers. I hope to goodness that my son never ends up in such a state!

I set about tidying him up; it was a job I had done often enough, though previously with elderly folk in care homes. I peeled off his clothes and gave him an old fashioned bed bath.

When it came to finding some cleanclothes for him there was a problem, there weren't any – so one of the nurses found an operating theatre gown, the traditional sort that you put your arms through at the front, then tie at the back. Then I went to collect a blanket from the linen cupboard to warm him up, but when I returned, he had disappeared. Frantically, I went in search and found him, still looking befuddled, by the reception desk. Where he thought he was going I couldn't imagine.

I led him back to his cubicle, wrapped him in the blanket, and

Sister, who had seen what had happened, asked me to stay with him until he settled. I looked at him through a mother's eye; a slightly built figure, with a gentle, almost innocent 'baby' face; fresh complexion, smooth-skinned and clean shaven. I was told he was twenty-years-old, but with his light-brown hair, and blue eyes, he looked a lot younger, barely out of childhood.

However, he wouldn't settle. One minute he would lie quietly on the trolley, the next he would get up and wander away. Fortunately, each time he went on one of his walks, I was able to coax him back to the cubicle without too much difficulty. Periodically, the nurses came in and examined him, taking his pulse, blood pressure, and assessing his mental state on what they called the Glasgow Coma Scale. But when I asked how he was, they simply said there had been no change, and that, indeed, is how it appeared to me. All the while he was awake, able to move about, didn't appear to be in pain or distress, but had this dull, confused expression on his face as he mumbled away, apparently in a world of his own.

I tried to engage him in conversation, I called him Sean, but he didn't respond. I asked where he lived and what he did for a living, but he didn't seem to hear what I was saying, and I never got a sensible reply. After a while, Sister said I could have a break, so I went to the canteen for a bite to eat, but within five minutes she sent word for me to come back. Apparently, as soon as I'd left the cubicle, the young man had again gone walkabout. This time he was found by the fire doors. I ended up having my mug of tea and sandwiches as I sat keeping an eye on him.

It was when I slipped off to spend a penny that the real problem arose. I was only away for a couple minutes, but when I got back to the cubicle, he'd disappeared again. I was just setting out in search of him when there was a shout from the far end of the department.

'Who's opened the fire doors, it's raining in and the wind is blowing wet leaves everywhere.'

There was a bang as the doors were slammed shut.

'No, no,' I cried, 'it will be the young man I've been watching.'

I ran to the doors and looked out just in time to see a ghostly white figure running barefoot and bare-buttocked across the field at the back of the hospital, his theatre gown flapping in the wind and rain. As fast as I could, I opened the doors and ran after him. Someone must have realised what was happening because almost at once a porter joined the pursuit.

At the far end of the field, there was a steep bank about thirty feet high that rose steeply to reach the dual carriageway, one of the main roads into the city.

When I caught up with him, the young man was half-way up the bank on his hands and knees, trying to reach the top but every time he gained a couple of feet he slid down again. With his bare feet in eighteen inches of slime and mud, he was making no progress at all. It was obvious that he was never going to make it to the top, but that didn't stop him trying and all the while he was getting ever muddier.

With the porter already on the way, I decided to wait for his assistance rather than attempt the climb myself, otherwise I should have ended up as filthy as he was. Occasionally, he fell face down and soon he was covered in mud from head to toe, his sodden theatre gown clinging to him. The only parts of his anatomy still free of the mud were his two white bare buttocks. I can't deny that the sight of him was amusing, and I was laughing out loud when eventually, exhausted by his efforts, he slid gently down to the bottom of the slope where the porter grabbed him, wrapped him in a blanket and returned him to the A & E department.

I was wet through, my hair hung in threads across my eyes, my dress was splattered with mud, and my shoes and stockings were filthy. Since it was nearly the end of my shift, Sister sent me off duty to go home to have a shower and change into some clean clothes. My dirty dress went straight into the washing machine.

It was only later I learned that when the police searched his car which had been left at the road side after the collision, they found a large quantity of drugs hidden under the seats.

Whether his 'confusion' was genuine or whether it was a charade to offer him the chance to escape to reclaim his stash of drugs, I never did discover.

A tangled tale

One Monday morning, my first task was to 'clerk in' three newly-admitted patients whose operations were planned for the next day. The first was Elsie Shawcross, an obese lady in her 70's, whose investigations in the outpatient clinic had revealed gallstones. Armed with her notes, I drew the screens around her bed, pulled a chair to her bedside, sat down, and introduced myself.

'You know,' she remarked, 'you doctors get more and more like policemen every day.'

'How so?' I replied.

'Well, you get younger and younger day by day. Do you know that the other day, when I was on my way to the shops, I walk you know as I think the exercise is good for me, well, it is, isn't it, and two bobbies pulled up in one of those Panda cars. Well, I looked them up and down, and neither of them looked old enough to have passed the driving test. I said to Liz, who was with me at the time, Liz is neighbour of mine, well I guess she's not just my neighbour, she's my very best friend, she'd do anything for you, you know, she really is very kind-hearted. Liz, I said, just look at those two young bobbies....'

'Yes,' I said, interrupting as gently as I could, 'they can look young, can't they? Now I need to ask you a few questions about the pain that's been troubling you. First of all, can you tell me precisely where you feel it?'

'There you are Doctor; you're just like that young bobby I was chatting to. He said he was busy and had to get on with his work. People these days don't seem to have the time to....

'Elsie,' I said, 'like that young policeman, I have a lot of jobs to get through this morning. Now tell me where you feel this pain of yours.'

'Well,' she said, 'the pain's in my belly, Doctor, really all over.'

'In every part of your belly?'

'Well, no,' she replied, 'mainly here.' With her left hand, she lifted up a pendulous right breast and pointed with her free hand to an area beneath her ribs.

'And how long does it last?'

'Well, it's there all the time,' came the reply.

'You mean throughout the entire day and night?'

'Well, no, not all the time, Doctor, but it's there a lot of the time.'

'Have you got it right now?'

She prodded her abdomen with her fingers, a look of concentration on her face.

'No,' she replied after careful consideration.

'Have you had it at all today?'

'No, not today, Doctor.'

'So when did you last have it?'

'Oh, some time ago now. I really can't remember.'

'And when you do get it, how long does it last?'

'Well, it's like a lightning flash, Doctor; it's gone in a second.'

I sighed. It seemed she would have me believe that this was a pain that was present all the time, but she couldn't remember when she last had it, and when it did occur, it only lasted for a second!

'And how severe is it when it comes?' I asked.

'Oh, Doctor,' she said, her eyes rolling to the ceiling, 'I can't tell you how bad it is.'

'How does it compare with labour pains?' I asked.

'Oh, far worse than that.'

'So what do you do when it comes?'

'Well, Doctor, as you know, woman's work is never done. I just get on with my jobs 'til it passes. Well, you have to, don't you?'

I wondered how many women managed to do their housework in the throes of labour. My difficulties increased when I tried to discover how long she had been experiencing pain.

'Oh, years and years, Doctor,' she said.

I tried to pin her down.

'Would you say weeks, months, or perhaps years?'

'Oh, a really long time, Doctor; years and years.'

'Could you say how long?'

'Well, I had an attack at our Billy's wedding and another when we had that holiday in Wales.'

'And how long ago was Billy married?'

'Oh, that's difficult to say, Doctor, quite some time because they've got the twins now.'

'And how old are the twins?'

'Oh, probably coming up two or three,' she said, 'but it took a long time for the babes to arrive. Our Billy's wife had to have some tests, you know. She went for some fancy new treatment in London. Then it took a long time for her to catch. Not that there's anything wrong with our Billy, you understand. He's a fine, strong, young man.'

I reverted to my original question.

'So how long do you think you've had the pain altogether?'

Unfortunately, she reverted to her original answer.

'Oh, years and years, Doctor!'

It was clear we were going round in circles and making little progress but I had to decide how to record these symptoms in the notes. In the end, I settled for *'Patient finds difficulty in giving details of the pain, states that it is present constantly, yet intermittently, is severe in intensity but doesn't interfere with housework, and has been present for a long time – probably many years!'*

Then I had to ask her about symptoms suggesting heart or lung problems that might interfere with the anaesthetic planned for her, and that took a further fifteen minutes.

Next came the physical examination, and I offered to get a chaperone. 'No need to bother, young man,' she said, 'when you've had as many babies as I have, you don't worry about such things.'

By the time I had completed the examination and written up her notes, over an hour had elapsed. I was mentally exhausted, and I still had two more patients to admit.

There was one consolation, though.

'Oh,' Elsie said, when I was gathering up my papers and preparing to move on, 'you're a nice young man. Perhaps we'll have time for a longer chat later!'

The Gentlefolk at St Ambrose

The St Ambrose Rest Home for Retired Gentlefolk was located in a suburb on the outskirts of a small market town in the Midlands. Originally the spacious home of a wealthy Victorian industrialist, it enjoyed generously proportioned grounds and was situated on what had once been a quiet street in a sleepy town. Since those days, however, the town had become popular with Birmingham commuters, the street had become congested, and cafes, shops, and offices had sprung up on both sides. The old mansion, now with a large modern extension, had become a care home for the elderly.

The residents, 36 in number, liked the title of 'Retired Gentlefolk', for that is how they regarded themselves. Privately owned and run, with weekly rates that were prohibitive, the home had a certain exclusivity that the residents valued.

They were mainly retired professional people of independent means, some living there of necessity because of infirmity, but others by choice. By and large, they were a contented bunch, the more able-bodied being happy to assist those with handicaps. Each resident had his or her own room and also enjoyed access to a number of communal rooms, dining room, library, television room, and a lounge in which a meeting of residents took place after lunch every Monday. It was unusual for there to be anything of great importance on the agenda, and it was generally regarded as a social event where it was decided which magazines should be bought for the library, or what was a suitable choice of a present for a retiring member of staff.

This week, however, Mary Cavendish, who chaired the meetings, had let it be known that she wanted every resident to attend as there was an important item to be discussed upon which urgent action was required. Mary was a sprightly 81-year-old spinster who had been the headmistress of a well-known private girl's prep school. At the appointed hour, she took her place at the end of the room, surveyed the retired gentlefolk who were present, and tapped her pen sharply on the table in front of her.

'Right,' she said, in the tone she used to attract the attention of a class of chattering school girls, 'I want you all to listen carefully because this week there's a matter of grave importance for us to discuss, something that affects the safety of all of us. It's about the traffic on High Street, and the danger we risk to life and limb every time we want to go to the shops.'

She went on to explain that during the previous week, she'd had an extremely frightening experience as she had crossed the road to visit the bank. 'As you know,' she continued, 'there's no safe place to cross. There are no lights, no zebra crossing, not even an island in the middle of the road to enable us to cross in two stages. With cars, lorries, and buses coming at you from both directions, many exceeding the speed limit, it's a death trap. We need to do something about it.'

She paused and was gratified to hear from the comments that followed, that her audience agreed wholeheartedly with her, indeed, several of them had become so fearful of crossing the road, they only ever visited the shops on the near side. When Mary asked what action should be taken, however, she was met with silence and a sea of blank faces; with one exception, they were indeed all 'gentle folk' not in the habit of creating waves.

She turned to Major Archie Burns, who at two in the afternoon had energy and enthusiasm, which faded as the day progressed and as the wine he imbibed with his evening meal took effect. The Major had led the protests when the management had tried to replace linen napkins with paper serviettes a couple of years before. What a fuss that had caused; but the Major's threat to arrange for outside caterers to deliver meals if the management didn't relent, had won the day.

He took a thoughtful puff on his cigar before replying. 'I think the answer is a pedestrian crossing,' he said, 'and that means approaching the local Council. What we need is a strongly-worded letter to the Highways Department stressing how the lack of a safe crossing exposes us to danger and limits our freedom to enjoy the local amenities.'

Mary agreed this was a splendid idea and said she would draft a letter to be approved the following week. Accordingly, the letter was drafted, approved, and posted. By return, a response was received stating that the matter would receive 'the attention of the appropriate subcommittee'. The residents waited... and waited... and waited.

Two months later, when nothing further had been heard from the Council, Mary decided that further action was required, and a plan began to form in her mind. She took the Major on one side and shared her ideas. The Major, always ready for a bit of fun, agreed that Mary's plan was just the stimulus needed to put pressure on the Council. He also felt it would provide the 'gentlefolk' of St Ambrose with an enjoyable afternoon's entertainment.

'To have the maximum impact, we need to get some publicity though,' the Major suggested. 'Let's see if the local radio station would be interested.'

'Or better still regional television,' Mary suggested.

Mary and the Major shared their plan with the other residents, and all were keen to participate. It promised to be an amusing diversion for them to enjoy. During the following weeks, the excitement in the Retirement Home reached fever pitch as the residents rehearsed their roles, initially in the lounge, then later, whenever the weather allowed, on the lawns. Finally, confident everyone had their equipment ready and were certain of the part they were to play in the little charade they had planned, they told the TV company where and when to be available.

***

In the middle of the afternoon the following week, Barry Webb was driving his delivery van southbound down the High Street when he saw a little old lady standing at the roadside, obviously waiting to cross. It was Mary. Nothing was coming in the opposite direction so, not being in any hurry and being a kind and considerate driver, he slowed, then stopped and waved to the lady to cross. Limping slowly with the help of two sticks, Mary stepped cautiously from the pavement. Reaching the middle of the road, she stopped to regain her breath, and to smile gratefully to Barry. Just as she set off again, an elderly gentleman drove his disability scooter off the pavement and followed in Mary's wake, and when he reached the middle of the road, a lady waving a white stick came behind.

The traffic was now held up in both directions, and Barry was beginning to get a little impatient. As he continued to watch this geriatric procession, two old men followed a few yards behind the lady with the white stick, both using walking frames. Then, a few yards behind them, came a white-haired woman struggling on crutches. Finally, a tall gentleman with a fine bristling moustache, proudly wearing his military medals on his chest, brought up the rear.

Barry's annoyance melted away when he realised he was witness to some sort of stunt, and he started to laugh, as did the driver at the front of the northbound queue. The drivers further back, unaware of what was causing the holdup, angrily sounded their horns. By this time, a sizeable crowd had collected, curious to see what was causing the congestion, and then laughing at the antics of these old folks. All the while, the scene was being filmed by a camera crew hidden on the first floor of the newsagents' shop.

When the Major got to the middle of the road, he paused to doff his cap and mouth his thanks to Barry, who put his van into gear with the intention of continuing his journey.

At that precise moment, though, Mary shouted to the Major, 'I'm afraid the bank's not open. We'll all have to go back.'

And so they did, the Major reversed his steps, followed by the woman on crutches, the two ladies with their walking frames, the blind lady, the man in the disability scooter and finally Mary, who again stopped to catch her breath in the middle of the road and smile her thanks to Barry.

***

That evening, the residents, having thoroughly enjoyed their day, all crowded around the television and were delighted to see themselves featured in the light-hearted item with which television presenters like to close their news programme. The soundtrack accompanying the film included an interview with Mary and the Major. It praised the initiative of the residents and criticised the Council for not responding to the needs of the elderly and infirm.

Within the week, the Council asked Mary exactly where she wished the pedestrian crossing to be placed, and within a month, it was installed.

Soccer Supporters Wrist

Gilbert and Sullivan maintained that 'a policeman's lot is not a happy one'. That may well be so, but it's a bed of roses when compared to the lot of the Casualty Officer who has to cope with everything that comes through the door, twenty-four-seven! One minute he or she will be relieving the pain of the retired bishop's gout, the next dealing with the drunk whose comatose state may be the result of the beer he has imbibed, or the head injury he sustained when falling down the steps of the pub. His next patient may be a child with a peanut stuck up his nose, or the victim of a stabbing who still has a knife sticking out of his chest.

I was working my way steadily through the patients attending the Casualty Department of Manchester's main hospital one Saturday evening in the 1970s, when three teenage boys arrived. Though I didn't realise it at the time, these lads were to have a significant influence on my attempts to climb the greasy promotion pole that is the surgical career ladder.

They had been watching the Manchester derby at the Old Trafford football ground. For Mancunians, this is one of the most important matches of the season. I can't remember now whether it was a cup match or a league match, and in any case, that's not relevant to the story. Nor can I recall whether it was City or United who won, not that that matters either, though I am sure it did to the boys at the time.

The three friends had four broken wrists between them, one left wrist, one right wrist, and one bilateral; he was the one who for the next six weeks would have the greatest difficulty wiping his bum.

These were the days before 'all seating' stadia were introduced. The youngsters had gone to the ground early and had taken their place behind one of the barriers that were used to break up the crowd. Each barrier had a concrete pillar at each end and these were joined along the top by a tubular steel bar. The lads watched the match with their hands resting, palms facing down, on the top of the bar, using it to raise themselves up should anyone standing in front of them block their view.

At a particularly exciting point in the match, the crowd behind them had surged forward down the steep slope of the terrace, crushing them against the barrier. This had forcibly overstretched their wrists, causing their injuries.

X-rays were taken, which confirmed that all four wrists were broken. Appropriate strapping and analgesia were arranged, and the boys were told to attend the fracture clinic the next morning, with their parents in attendance, to have the fractures reduced.

At the time, busy as I was in the Casualty Department, I gave little thought to the matter, but later I began to wonder whether this was recognised as a mechanism of injury. I knew that most wrist injuries were caused by falling onto an outstretched hand. People slip and put their hands out to break their fall. There's always a glut of such injuries whenever there is snow or ice on the ground. If wrist injuries watching football matches was something that hadn't previously been recognised, maybe I could write a report and get it published in a surgical journal. If so, it would certainly look good on my CV.

It seemed logical that such injuries were most likely to occur when the grounds were full, so I rang the sports editor of the local newspaper. I needed to know the dates on which the attendance at football matches was greatest; arbitrarily, I suggested in excess of sixty thousand. The editor was most obliging and gave me access to their sports archives in return for a commitment to write a feature article for them should my research prove fruitful.

Subsequently, armed with the dates when the crowd was close to capacity, I was able to review the records of patients who attended Casualty within 24 hours of these matches and, lo and behold, I found four further cases. All were teenage boys!

The article, when it was published in an orthopaedic journal, was a winner. Entitled *'Soccer Supporter's Wrist'*, I placed it prominently on my CV.

I was delighted. The more competitive the medical specialty, and surgery is particularly cut-throat, the greater the need for a trainee to stand out from the crowd. It wasn't enough to keep your nose clean, pass the appropriate exams, and get a good reference from your boss; you needed to publish articles in learned journals and read papers to academic societies. A 'publish or perish' attitude had developed, and regrettably this had led to an environment where trainees often undertook research for the wrong reasons. Little did I know that the article I had published was to lead me into a fateful game of snakes and ladders, initially in helping me advance my career before causing a disastrous slide.

Buoyed with this success and wishing to further enhance my CV, I applied to make a presentation to the British Upper and Lower Limb Society (known as BULL for short). I did this more in hope than expectation and was therefore pleasantly surprised when it was accepted for their annual conference. I suspect the Society thought a short talk entitled *Soccer Supporter's Wrist* would offer light relief amongst all the more worthy academic presentations. The meeting of the Society was to be held the following month in London.

I know our capital city has much to recommend it, and that it is a popular destination for thousands of overseas visitors, but I confess that it's not my favourite city. It evokes in me, memories of sleepless nights in stuffy third rate hotels prior to nerve-wracking examinations. Nonetheless, I knew these were experiences I had to endure if I was to advance my career.

I spent much time preparing for the event, seeking advice from my consultant, preparing slides and practising delivering my talk in a clear and confident voice. I was allocated a ten-minute slot, and my instructions were to speak for a maximum of six minutes and be prepared to answer questions for the rest of the time. There was to be a system of lights displayed on the lectern; green indicating all was well, a warning light of amber meaning I had just one minute left, and a red light which meant shut up immediately, because in fifteen seconds the microphone will be switched off!

In the days leading up to the event, I spent many evenings ensuring that my timing was spot on. My main concern, though, was the four minutes allowed for questions; the audience would mainly be consultant orthopaedic surgeons; as a junior doctor, would I be able to answer them? Finally, as well prepared as I was able to be, I travelled to London.

The symposium was spread over three days, my presentation being scheduled for the Saturday morning, so I travelled to London by train early on the Friday. My plan was to spend the day in the hall where the presentations were given, getting my bearings, and observing how other speakers coped with the light system on the lectern. One or two speakers were unaware of the length of their talks and, as a result, they were summarily terminated in mid-sentence. But the rigidity with which the rule was applied, appeared to depend on the seniority of the speaker. One overseas professor managed to speak for the best part of thirty minutes before the chairman politely suggested that the meeting was running a little behind schedule!

Saturday morning dawned, and it became apparent that many delegates had gone home early; there were, however, still twenty or thirty people in the hall for the first session in the morning. I was pleased. I would have been far more nervous had the hall been packed.

Returning to the hall after the coffee break, I was amazed to find that only a single individual remained. He was a fresh-faced young man who looked no older than I was. Presuming that folk were just being a little slow returning after the break, I sat and waited for them to resume their places, but a couple of minutes later the projectionist, sounding rather irritated at the delay, instructed me to start my talk.

It was a great anti-climax to find myself talking to rows and rows of empty seats, but I consoled myself with the thought that my CV would still boast of this presentation, and at any subsequent job interview, no one would know that I'd spoken to an audience of one.

My six minutes completed, there being no questions from my one supporter, I left the stage. As I turned to leave, I thanked him for listening.

'Oh, please don't go,' he said, 'I'm the last speaker!'

***

At future job interviews, the interviewing panel, in those days invariably male, couldn't resist asking about *Soccer Supporter's Wrist*. It enabled me to talk at length on a topic with which I was fully conversant and in which the panel was genuinely interested. It left them little time to quiz me on more awkward matters. At one interview, I wondered aloud whether such injuries might occur at rugby matches. It transpired that two of the panel held debentures at Twickenham and they started discussing the question between themselves whilst I simply sat there listening. The whole interview passed in a flash, and I was offered the post for which I had applied without any other subject being raised.

A couple of years later, however, my luck changed, and I ended up cursing the day those three lads had entered my life. At this particular interview, the panel consisted of a number of doctors but also a representative of the University, a Professor of Law.

'Well, it certainly makes an interesting article,' the Professor said when I'd informed him how the injuries had been sustained, 'and I presume you reported your findings to the Football Association?'

'The Football Association, sir?'

'Yes, the Football Association.'

'No, I didn't, sir,' I said, wondering why he should expect the Football Association to be involved.

'Perhaps you informed the police?'

My silence and the expression on my face indicated to the Professor that I was at a loss to understand the question.

The Professor frowned. 'What was the purpose of recording this injury?'

'I thought it would be of interest, sir.'

'And look good on your CV, perhaps.' This was spoken as an accusation rather than as a comment.

I couldn't deny this. Everyone in the hospital service recognised that in a highly competitive speciality such as surgery, the stronger the CV, the better the chance of promotion. Surely the Professor, with his academic background, would acknowledge this.

'Look,' he said sternly, 'you have been observant enough to identify a cause of injury at football matches, but surely you must realise that injuries of this kind will continue to occur unless the design of the grounds or the management of crowds changes. The Football Association and the police are responsible for public safety at football matches, yet you've done nothing to inform them. How many more broken wrists have there been at football matches, how many more boys have suffered pain and disability since you identified the problem?'

Without waiting for a reply, the Professor added to my discomfort. 'Have you taken the trouble to find out if such injuries are occurring at rugby grounds too, perhaps at Twickenham, where large crowds gather for rugby internationals?'

I had to admit I hadn't, despite the possibility of injuries at rugby matches having been raised in that previous interview.

The Professor then proceeded to give me a short but formal lecture on the reasons for research, stressing that advances in medical knowledge should immediately be followed by consideration of the way in which patients may be benefitted. Then he looked me straight in the eye.

'The reason for research is not simply to publish an article in a medical journal so that it looks good on your curriculum vitae.'

There was a short silence, and gloomily, I reflected on what had happened. A discussion on wrist injuries ought to have been my strong suit, an opportunity to present myself as an astute observer, a diligent researcher with an active mind. Instead, it had turned into a disaster, merely revealing my selfish motive for the study and a desire for self-aggrandisement. I left the interview with my head down and, no, I didn't get the job.

The Failed Vasectomy Operation

Don's heart sank when he saw the letter sitting on his desk. The envelope was of high quality; it bore a first-class stamp and had a London postmark. In his experience, such letters rarely brought good news! Apprehensively, he opened it. The notepaper was thick and expensive, certainly not the sort used in the health service! He read the address on the top of the page. It caused a shiver to pass down his back.

> Williams, Cummings and Lane. 'Solicitors.
> Specialists in medical negligence.'
> 25 Chancery Lane, London

With an increasing sense of foreboding Don read the letter:

Dear Mr Fraser,

Re. Frederick Makin

We write to inform you that we act on behalf of the above-named client upon whom you undertook a vasectomy operation. This operation was undertaken in a negligent fashion, as a result of which Mr Makin has fathered a child. Further details will be forwarded to you in due course. It is expected that the damages will be in the region of £90,000.

Yours etc
Harvey Lane

Don's first reaction was one of anger. He had been a consultant for twenty years, during which time he had devoted himself to his patients, and to the health service. How dare they accuse him of negligence? He worked long hours; he was 'on-call' for emergencies every fourth night, and every fourth weekend; and he was regularly reprimanded by his wife for putting his patients before his home life.

And how on earth did they arrive at the figure of £90,000? To repeat the vasectomy operation, if indeed it had failed, couldn't possibly justify such a sum in compensation. And if Mr Makin - whomever he was - had the joy of a baby in the house, he damn well ought to be grateful. Don and his wife had always wanted a family but had not been so fortunate.

Even as these thoughts raced through his head, he already had an idea as to the cause of the problem. He was probably being sued, not because the operation had failed, but because the patient hadn't been warned that failure was a possibility. These were the early days of male sterilisation, and a standard *'consent for vasectomy'* form had yet to be produced.

Within a couple of days, on reviewing Frederick Makin's medical records, his fears were confirmed; there was indeed no written record that he had been warned the operation might fail, and that he might father a child.

Three weeks later, a further letter from Williams Cummings and Lane arrived, detailing their justification for the £90,000 claim. The inventory included everything from nappies and a pram when their latest arrival was a baby, toys and a bike as he grew up, trips to the cinema and driving lessons when he reached the age of 17 and food, clothes and holidays throughout!! They argued that had Mr and Mrs Makin known the operation might fail, they would not have had it performed; they would have practised an alternative form of contraception. But now they had produced another child; he was entitled to the same benefits in his life as his older siblings.

Now considerably alarmed, Don rang his medical insurance company. He was relieved to learn that not only would they support him with legal advice; they would also cover the damages should the case be lost. Strangely however, though he was reassured that his own money was not at risk, he remained deeply hurt and angry by the accusation of negligence. He regarded it as an unjustifiable stain on his reputation.

The question that particularly troubled him was the legal test upon which the court would make its judgement. This was whether giving a warning that the operation might fail, was the accepted medical practice at the time the vasectomy was performed. If it was, the case was lost! Don thought it wasn't usual to give such a warning but the medical insurance company were less sure. A meeting was arranged for the matter to be discussed.

'The problem,' the legal advisor began, 'is that we are reasonably certain that an out-of-court settlement could be reached at a figure of about £30,000. The danger, of course, is that if the matter is contested in court, and we lose, then the damages will be the full £90,000, with costs to pay on top of that.'

Don felt that settling out of court too readily, simply encouraged others to follow suit and that, in the long run, it was cheaper to contest the matter. He argued that if a few claimants lost their cases, received no compensation, and had to pay costs, then there would be fewer spurious claims in the future. The truth was, although he wouldn't admit it, that his pride was at stake; the accusation of his alleged 'negligence' still rankled. Eventually, albeit with some reluctance, the insurance company backed down, and a date for the court case was fixed.

As the day of the trial approached, Don became increasingly anxious and moody. At home, he was irritable and found difficulty sleeping. At work, he began to lose his concentration and his confidence. He wondered how he would cope when cross-examined by some silver-tongued barrister under oath. He spent long hours in the medical library researching the subject. Certainly, he found a number of instances where surgeons had reported vasectomy failures, but at the time of Mr Makin's operation, no recognised professional body had formally recommended warning patients of this complication. It seemed to him that the outcome of the court case would be a matter of opinion. It could go either way. He also realised that an out-of-court settlement now looked the better option, and thought perhaps he should not have argued his point of view with the insurance company quite so forcibly. He rang the insurers to tell them so.

'Too late now, I'm afraid,' came the reply. 'A date for the trial has been set, a judge has been appointed and briefed, and in any case, if we were to make an offer to the claimant now, it would certainly be refused. They would recognise that we were conceding defeat.'

A couple of days later, as Don got more and more concerned, one of his pals, a surgeon in a neighbouring hospital, rang him. He sounded cheerful.

'Hi, Don. I've got some interesting news for you,' he said. 'I operated today on an old patient of yours, a chap called Makin. He told me he was making a claim against you. Obviously, I pricked up my ears and probed for more details. I thought you would be interested to know that the operation I was doing was a repeat vasectomy.'

'So....?' Don enquired, not understanding the significance of this news.

'Well, don't you see? His legal argument is that had he known his first vasectomy operation might fail, he would never have had it done. Well, from his own experience, he *does* now know the operation can fail, yet despite that, he's had it repeated. He's undermined his own argument. His case against you completely collapses.'

There was silence for a moment while Don considered this new information.

'Why so it does,' Don said, as a huge smile of relief lit up his face. 'I'll phone the medical insurance company at once. Thank you so much.'

Then he rang his wife and told her the good news.

'Well, thank goodness for that,' she said. 'What a great relief. Now perhaps you'll go back to being your old self again.'

Thought for the day

If it's not written down, it didn't happen.

Unknown

Fiddling the figures

'Too many chiefs and not enough Indians' has been a common criticism of the Health Service for many years. Certainly, those at the coalface, if I may be allowed to mix my metaphors, frequently complain that there are too many managers and insufficient doctors, nurses, and paramedics, a theme that has frequently been picked up in the popular press.

Working as a consultant on a surgical unit at the time, Bernard Wilkins was therefore delighted to hear at a committee meeting, of a Government initiative to increase the proportion of clinical staff in the hospital. Great, he thought, a chance to improve staffing levels on the ward.

Bernard therefore, raised the matter under 'Any other Business' addressing his question to the Chief Executive.

'Yes', he was assured, 'such a directive has indeed been issued by the Department of Health; the ratio of clinical staff to managerial staff is to be adjusted in favour of the clinical staff. All hospitals are required to become compliant within a fixed time period.'

'And how long is this fixed period?' Bernard asked.

'Six months'.

'And are we compliant at present?'

'No, we aren't. We have some work to do to address the problem.'

Bernard was delighted. Here was a chance to bolster the staff on the wards.

During the next couple of weeks, with the help of his Nursing Sisters, he wrote a formal business case to increase the complement of nurses by two on each of the surgical wards and submitted it to the Chief Executive. Working on the assumption that his request would not be granted in full, and certain that others would be hoping to take advantage of this opportunity, he added a request for a theatre nurse and theatre orderly as well. His submission was acknowledged, so he sat back and waited expectantly.

Three months passed. Then another three and still Bernard had heard nothing, so at the next meeting, again under 'Any Other Business', he asked for a progress report.

'I'm pleased to say that the requirements of the NHS Directive have now been met,' the Chief Executive announced.

'You mean we are now compliant and have improved the ratio of clinical staff to managers?'

'That's correct.'

Bernard was puzzled, his application for more nurses hadn't been granted, he wasn't aware that any new clinical staff had been appointed elsewhere in the hospital, and there seemed to be just as many managers as before.

'So how many extra nurses do we now employ?'

'We didn't find it necessary to increase their number.'

'So presumably we now have some additional paramedical staff: physios, dieticians, or healthcare assistants?'

'No.'

'In that case, you must have reduced the number of managers.'

The CEO was starting to look a bit shifty. 'Not necessarily,' he said.

'Well, if you haven't increased the number of clinical staff, and haven't reduced the number of managers, how can we be compliant with the Directive now, if we weren't before?' Bernard demanded.

'We decided to classify the consultants' secretaries as clinical staff!'

Is Having Sex the same as Making Love?

With his consultant away for a few days, Paul was teaching the medical students. It was a task he enjoyed, but thanks to the short notice he had been given, he hadn't been able to prepare himself as thoroughly as he would have liked.

Without exception, the students were intelligent, but they differed greatly in their ability to communicate with patients. Some had a natural empathy. Patients opened their hearts quickly and easily to them, and, as a result, they found little difficulty in eliciting their patient's symptoms. Other students however, found talking to patients difficult, perhaps because English was not their first language, maybe because of their natural reserve, or occasionally due to a superior or haughty manner. An essential task for their tutors was to observe the interaction between student and patient and to guide and advise as necessary.

Paul gathered the students round the bed of a rather deaf octogenarian who came from Pontefract in Yorkshire. On this occasion, it was Sunil Solanki's turn to demonstrate his ability to take a patient's history. Sunil had been nicknamed 'Sunny' because of his cheerful disposition and ready smile.

'Now, Sunny,' Paul began, 'Mr Howell has a problem with his bowels. I would like you to ask him to describe his symptoms.'

Paul turned to the other students. 'The rest of you should listen carefully, and be prepared to chip in and make comments – but only if you feel it's something important. Right, away you go, Sunny.'

Sunny approached the patient somewhat nervously. 'Good morning, Mr Howell,' he said politely.

'What's that you said, young man?' the patient shouted.

'I said, Good morning, Mr Howell.'

'Aye, that's me, 'owell's me name.'

'I hear you have trouble shitting,' Sunil continued.

'Ouch,' interrupted Miss Croft. 'I don't think you should use the word *shitting*. Many patients, especially ladies, would be most upset.'

Sunny looked puzzled. 'But *shitting* is the same as *crapping*, I'm told. I have a doctor friend who is telling me all about English as it is spoken, and that's what he says.'

'Yes, that's true,' Paul explained, 'but *shitting* and *crapping* are both rude words – not words to be used in polite society, and certainly not with patients. Were you taught any other words for the act of moving the bowels?'

'Yes,' Sunny replied as if he had suddenly remembered. He turned again to Mr Howell. 'Are you having trouble with your ha-ha?'

'With what young man?' Mr Howell yelled, a cupped hand to his ear.

'With ha-ha?'

The patient turned to Paul. 'I 'ope 'e's not laughing at me. I'll not stand for that.'

'No, certainly not,' Paul said, laying a reassuring hand on Mr Howell's arm. 'Sunny, I'm afraid there are lots of words in English for our various bodily functions. *Ha-ha* is a phrase sometimes used by children. *Number twos* and *having a poo* are other expressions, but again only used by youngsters. They're not words you would use to an adult. *Moving your bowels* is probably as good a phrase as any, though the proper verb is *defaecation*. Now start again.'

Now, both confused and embarrassed, Sunny tried again.

'You are having trouble with your defaecation?' he said, raising his voice.

'Beg pardon, young man?'

'Trouble with your defaecation?' Sunny repeated even louder.

'I don't know 'owt about 'defee whatever that is'. And there's no need to shout, young man; I may be a bit daft, but I'm not deaf.'

At Paul's suggestion, Sunny asked if Mr Howell was having trouble with his bowels.

'My balls did you say.' Mr Howell shouted back. 'Let me tell you, lad, I've only got one ball. I lost t'other one years ago. Jerry shot it off in that little scrap we had with 'err 'itler! But I've found that one works just as well as two, if you know what I mean,' Mr Howell replied with a dirty laugh while giving Sunny a dig in the ribs, which surprised and mystified him.

It took the best part of thirty minutes for Sunny to draw out the story of Mr Howell's bowel problems. Having had a regular bowel habit previously, he now had a constant desire to go to the toilet, but when he went, he passed little more than a small amount of slimy stool mixed with blood. Paul hoped that as a result of the session, the students would remember the significance of a change in bowel habit and the presence of blood in the stool. Unfortunately, Mr

Howell had a tumour in his rectum.

Later, back in the tutorial room, Sunny again raised the subject of colloquial English. 'If *number twos* is the same as *defaecation*,' he asked, 'does *number one* mean *pissing*?'

'Yes, it does,' Paul explained, 'but *pissing* is also a rude word. *Having a pee* or *spending a penny* are better phrases. More often, you would ask a patient if he has trouble passing water. The formal medical term, of course, is *micturition*.'

'If number one is having a pee and number two is moving the bowels, what is number three? Is it fucking?'

Paul couldn't help but laugh. 'Sunny, you need to learn which words to use in different circumstances, or you're going to find yourself in some embarrassing situations. There isn't a *number three,* and since the number system is used by young children, they wouldn't know about *number three*, even if it was what you suggest. In any case, the word *fucking* is extremely crude. *Humping*, *shagging* and *screwing* are almost as bad, but you might just get away with *rumpy-pumpy'*. If you wanted to ask a patient about sexual relations, you would speak of *having intercourse* or *having sex.*'

'Another expression would be *making love*,' Miss Croft added quietly, catching Paul's eye and offering him a coy smile as she did so.

'Sunny,' Paul continued, ignoring the interruption despite it having caused his heart to skip a beat and his concentration to falter, 'I fear the friend who helped you with your English has been having a laugh at your expense. I suggest you ask one of the other students to write down the terms used for bodily functions and list those that are acceptable and those that are not. Now, if there are no more questions, I think....'

Suddenly, he was interrupted by the emergency tone emitted by his bleep. 'Cardiac Arrest... Surgical 5 female ward. Cardiac Arrest.... Surgical 5 female.'

Paul heard the message and dashed to the ward with mixed feelings. He didn't like cardiac arrests, never feeling totally confident of his ability to cope – but at least it stopped him thinking about the remark made by the attractive Karen Croft.

The Celtic Supporter

'I canna' understand the lad. There's many a bonny Scots lass would have wed him. He'll nae be happy with a Sassenach wife, pretty though she may be. But he's made his own bed. He'll be the one to lie in it!'

The words were spoken by Jimmy McMillan, a Glaswegian milkman. He was a diabetic who needed insulin injections to control his sugar levels. He had travelled south to attend his brother's wedding. With his wiry stature and a shock of red hair, he was extremely patriotic. He couldn't understand why his brother should choose to take an English girl as his bride, when there were plenty of lovely girls in Scotland his brother could have married.

Nonetheless, this had not prevented him from enjoying the lunchtime reception that followed the marriage, or the drinks that flowed freely thereafter. When the wedding festivities were over, Jimmy and a few of his mates drifted to one of the local pubs and continued to celebrate late into the evening. Then disaster struck.

He had been nursing a groin hernia for several months and was waiting to have it repaired at the Royal Infirmary in Glasgow. In the meantime, he had been advised that should the rupture become painful and swollen; he should lie down and ease the swelling back into the abdominal cavity where it belonged. He had undertaken this manoeuvre successfully on a number of occasions, but in recent weeks, pushing the hernia back had become increasingly difficult.

When the rupture had become swollen after the wedding, he hadn't felt much pain, the beer he'd consumed having acted as an anaesthetic. He had therefore ignored it and continued to celebrate with his friends. Now, stand, sit, or lie, he couldn't persuade the swelling to return to the abdomen, and he was in agony. His friends had been thoughtful enough to deposit him in the casualty department of the nearest hospital but had then continued on their merry way.

Standing scarcely five feet in height, Jimmy was slimly built with a jockey's physique. However, the most striking thing about his appearance was not his height or ginger locks, but his upper body. As a milkman, he had a physical job. It required upper body strength to load heavy crates every day onto the back of his milk float, but he also undertook weight training in the gym and had fought with considerable success as an amateur boxer. His chest and shoulder muscles, especially his pectoral muscles, were remarkably well-developed. He was proud of his physique and consequently wore his shirt with the top three buttons open, displaying his muscles to maximum effect. A thick gold chain, bearing a large gold medallion encircled his neck, enhancing the appearance. But most noticeable of all, was his tattoo. Across his upper chest, in bold letters two inches tall, there was emblazoned a single word 'CELTIC'.

When Jimmy dropped his pants to allow John, the surgical registrar to examine him, the hernia was an impressive sight. The size of an orange, it was tense and painful. Jimmy clearly needed to be admitted. John assumed he would have emergency surgery that night; that was the standard practice for such cases. But Mr Khan, the senior registrar on the surgical unit, surprised him by suggesting that the operation be deferred until the next day. He was afraid that Jimmy's drinking might have upset his diabetes and wanted his blood sugar levels to be monitored. He also had a trick up his sleeve. He asked John to sedate Jimmy, to relieve his pain and then get him to sleep on a couch with his head well below the level of his feet.

A couple of hours later, John reviewed the situation and thanks to the sedation found Jimmy to be pain-free. Mr Khan's plan had worked like a dream, and John was now able to reduce the hernia without difficulty. Jimmy was delighted and announced his intention to leave the department forthwith and to return to the accommodation he and his pals had rented for the night. This course of action was clearly unwise. He had been sedated, his diabetes was poorly controlled, and if he stayed where he was, he would have his hernia repaired within the next couple of days.

An intemperate Scot, Jimmy announced that he wasn't at all sure he wanted *'to be butchered by any old English surgeon'* saying he preferred Mr Angus McDonald to operate on him in Glasgow. However, when reminded he was currently losing time off work, didn't know how quickly his hernia would be repaired in Glasgow and, in the meantime, was at risk of further episodes of pain, he changed his mind.

Although pint-sized, Jimmy had a big personality. He was quick-witted, cheeky, indeed cocky at times. The nurses found it impossible to resist the temptation to chide him about the state of Scottish football. England had recently won the World Cup, and the impressive tattoo on his chest invited comment. But Jimmy was in no way abashed and defended his Celtic heroes vehemently.

'Aye,' he said. 'England may have done well in the World Cup, but you watch out for Celtic in the next few years. You can keep your Arsenals, Tottenhams and Manchester Uniteds. Celtic will be beating them all within a couple of years. We've a new manager and a string of young players, all of them local lads; Tommy Gemmell, Billy McNeill and Jimmy Johnstone. Mark those names well; you'll hear a lot about them in the next few years. Two years ago, Celtic won every competition they entered, and that included the European Cup. That's when I had this tattoo done on my chest.'

He stuck out his chest to display the tattoo in its full glory. 'My father was a Celtic man before me, I shall be a Celtic man 'til the day I die, and if I ever have kids, they will be Celtic supporters too.'

'I thought Rangers were the only decent football team in Glasgow,' John said to tease him. It would be an understatement to say his response was uncharitable. It was, in fact, unprintable.

***

Jimmy was entirely at ease on the ward whilst waiting for his operation. He settled into the hospital routine without difficulty, never missing an opportunity to 'chat up' the nurses, with whom he became quite a favourite. Since there was no reason for him to be confined to his bed, he took it upon himself to perform his own ward rounds.

He thoroughly enjoyed talking to the other patients, criticising whichever team they happened to support, belittling English football in general and regaling anyone prepared to listen of the exploits of his beloved Celtic football team. He was constantly cheerful, with an outgoing and optimistic personality. He made himself useful by helping the nurses to serve meals to bed-bound patients and happily assisted in tidying away the trays and dishes afterward. He ran errands for less-mobile patients and visited the hospital shop from time to time on their behalf.

He met Mr Willoughby Scott, the hospital's senior surgeon, the next day during the consultant's ward round. Although Jimmy was sitting with his pyjama jacket widely unbuttoned, flaunting his gold medallion, his rippling pectoral muscles and his CELTIC tattoo, Mr Scott made no comment, much to Jimmy's disappointment. As he commented afterward, '*I thought it was those of us from north of the border that were supposed to be the dour ones.*'

***

When the day scheduled for his operation arrived, Jimmy objected violently when told to remove the gold chain and medallion that were so prominently displayed around his neck. He only agreed, when it was explained that the diathermy machine used during surgery to coagulate bleeding vessels, applied an electric current to the body, which would cause a burn at the site of his chain. This would not only be painful but would also cause a scar and disfigure his tattoo.

A surgeon's time is divided more or less equally between the wards, the clinic and the operating theatre, but for most, it is the time spent in theatre that they find the most enjoyable. As John became more experienced and his technical ability developed, he too, gained the greatest satisfaction from operating. He was conscious, of course, that operating on a fellow human being was a huge responsibility. Patients entrust themselves to their surgeon. They rely on his knowledge of anatomy, his understanding of their disease, his experience and his manual dexterity to treat them in an intensely personal way. The surgeon must be meticulous in everything he does, since his skill, or lack of it, determines the patient's outcome. A successful operation can save a patient's life. Failure may lead to his death. There is much truth in the old surgical adage that '*a surgeon needs the eye of a hawk, the hands of a lady and the heart of a lion*'.

John's assistant was a house officer called Richard, a pleasant young man who retained a boyish sense of humour and when he saw Jimmy's impressive tattoo, he smiled and said, 'I think we could have some fun with that.'

Fortunately, the procedure went according to plan and no particular problems were encountered. John found the defect in the muscles through which the hernia had protruded, he was able to close it with strong sutures and, fifty minutes later, he was applying a dressing to the wound.

Whilst undertaking the surgery, concentrating intently, John had

55

been a member of a close-knit team of anaesthetist, nurses, and technicians, all working with a common aim. Jimmy had experienced a great deal of discomfort from his hernia. It had interfered with his job, and the episode that had resulted in his admission to the hospital had been life-threatening. Provided he now made a good recovery, he would be cured, and it had been John's surgery that had achieved this. The warm glow induced by successfully completing an operation was like a drug; it was addictive.

John was aware, of course, that surgery could induce other emotions. There were times when concerns over his own ability and limited experience caused him anxiety. But he was still at a stage when he could call for assistance if problems arose. It was reassuring to know that the final responsibility for the patient was not his. He often wondered though, what it must feel like to be the consultant, the most senior member of the team, the one who 'carried the can'.

As the theatre sheets were removed, Jimmy's tattooed chest was again exposed, and as he was lifted onto a trolley and wheeled to the recovery area, Richard followed, a twinkle in his eye.

'I'm just going to have a look at that tattoo,' he said over his shoulder.

***

The next day, when John went to review Jimmy on the ward, he was surprised to find a gaggle of nurses at his bedside. He went to investigate. He needed to reassure himself there wasn't a problem, either with the operation he had performed or with Jimmy's diabetes. However, the nurses appeared relaxed; indeed, they were teasing him about his Glaswegian football team. Jimmy was sitting in bed, enjoying being the centre of attention. As usual, his pyjama jacket was unbuttoned, displaying his physique; the gold chain and medallion having been restored to their rightful place, alongside the tattoo of which he was so proud.

On closer inspection, the cause of the nurses' good humour was apparent. Whilst Jimmy had been anaesthetized somebody, John presumed it to be Richard, had taken liberties with the tattoo using an indelible marker pen. Unable to see the upper part of his own chest, Jimmy was happily oblivious to Richard's handiwork. The result of the alteration was undeniably amusing, but John felt a twinge of anxiety. Mr Scott was not known for his sense of humour. He held traditional views about a patient's right to be treated with respect and dignity. There could be unpleasant consequences if he took exception to this light-hearted prank.

Over the next couple of days, the tattoo caused much amusement, and, as a result, Jimmy became something of a celebrity. The ward staff commented on it whenever they dispensed his pain killers or dressed his wound, as did other therapists, such as dieticians and physiotherapists. As word of the tattoo spread on the hospital grapevine, porters went out of their way to pass Jimmy's bed. They chatted to him about the Celtic football team, but nobody informed him that his tattoo had been compromised. Jimmy loved his football. He knew a great deal about English clubs, including the two first division sides in the city, and there was much genial banter about the relative merits of teams north and south of the border. However, the conspiracy of silence amongst all who spoke with him continued, and he lapped up the attention, in complete ignorance of the real reason for the interest in Celtic.

When the time came for the next consultant ward round, there was a general concern that Mr Scott might '*let the cat out of the bag*', and, that if he did, Jimmy, despite his good nature, would not be amused. He might prove to have a short Scottish fuse and cause a scene or even make a formal complaint. In particular, Mr Khan was afraid Mr Scott would consider that making one of his patients the butt of a joke was disrespectful, and that Richard would be punished.

When the consultant arrived, Mr Khan reminded him of the Scottish milkman whom he had met a few days earlier; the one who had been reluctant to entrust himself to an English surgeon. He proceeded to confess that liberties had been taken with his tattoo but that, to date, the patient was unaware an alteration had been made. Mr Scott listened carefully but didn't ask in what way the tattoo had been changed; nor did he request the name of the individual responsible. However, frowning ominously, he gravely reminded the team that patients should be treated with the respect they would expect themselves if the situation were reversed. He added he would have to see the tattoo before deciding what action would be appropriate.

In due course, the team arrived at Jimmy's bed. Jimmy had his pyjama jacket open to the waist as usual. Although Mr Scott could not fail to see Richard's graffiti, he made no comment upon it but, in a manner unfamiliar to him, he enquired diligently about the patient's progress. He inspected the wound and even looked at the diabetic chart to check that Jimmy's sugar levels were satisfactory, which, fortunately they were.

'I'm pleased to see you're making good progress,' the consultant said to Jimmy, 'but you will need to stay with us until you become mobile. I'll review you again in a couple of days, and decide when you can go home. All in all, though, things are going well.'

'Aye, Doctor,' Jimmy replied. 'We have good healing flesh north of the border.'

John was reminded of one of Mr Scott's favourite anecdotes. *'If a wound heals well', he would say, 'the patient takes the credit and comments on his good healing flesh. But if it fails to heal or becomes infected, the surgeon is deemed responsible and the patient asks, 'What's gone wrong with your wound, Doctor?''*

Mr Scott started to lead his entourage towards the next bed, but then appeared to change his mind. He turned and spoke again to Jimmy.

'So you decided to trust an English surgeon after all, did you?'

Jimmy faced with the consultant and his retinue of doctors and nurses, was more subdued than usual. He answered politely.

'Och, I was only joking with the young doctors. I'm grateful to you for doing the operation. If I'd gone back to Glasgow, I shouldna' been able to work and would still be awaiting my operation. But now, thanks to you, I've put it behind me. I'm feeling grand and raring to go.'

'So, you approve of the way we do things in England, do you?' Mr Scott asked.

There was a moment's pause. Was he about to spill the beans?

'Oh, definitely,' said Jimmy.

'Well I hope nothing happens before you go home to make you change your mind.'

Mr Scott, having spent more time chatting to this one patient than he normally did on an entire ward round, smiled and moved on. There was a collective sigh of relief from the doctors and nurses accompanying him. Clearly, he had decided that Richard's handiwork was no more than a bit of harmless fun.

It was inevitable that Jimmy would eventually become suspicious that so many people stopped, grinned, and made comments about the Celtic football team when they passed his bed. Slowly but surely, a doubt built in his mind until finally, he was forced to the conclusion that something must be wrong with his tattoo. Ultimately, there came the moment when he could bear the uncertainty no longer. Unable to see the upper part of his chest and not possessing a hand mirror, he got out of bed and limped slowly down the ward, clutching his wound to reduce the pain that resulted from movement. In the washroom, he stood in front of the long mirror. To his horror, he read Richard's handiwork. The tattoo read 'CELTIC 0 - RANGERS 4'

Afterwards, John reflected it was episodes such as this that enlivened hospital life and made the long hours, hard work and disrupted nights tolerable. In years to come, it would become unacceptable to have such a joke at a patient's expense. It might be considered a physical assault on their person or judged to be psychologically distressing. It could result in a demand for counselling or in legal action and compensation! The European Court of Human Rights might even express concerns about racial abuse, given all the banter there had been about Scotland and Scottish football teams.

As it was Jimmy, after a few expletives and curses about the staff in general and about Richard in particular (after he had discovered who was responsible) saw the funny side of the escapade and continued to enjoy his celebrity status. As before, he wore his pyjama jacket open, and flaunted his physique, medallion, and tattoo but only after he had persuaded the nurses to remove the offending extra letters with methylated spirits!

Family Planning

Dr Julie Smith was coming to the end of a busy family planning clinic. During a long and tiring day, she had discussed the merits of contraceptive pills, caps, condoms, coils injections, and implants so frequently, so repetitively, that she feared the disenchantment she felt with her job might become apparent to her patients, or clients, as her boss insisted they be called. Five years previously, she had aspired to become a consultant gynaecologist but, now married, she was forced to settle for work that paid the mortgage, enabled her to run her home, and care for her two young children, but gave her little job satisfaction. In the course of the afternoon, she had seen silly girls, sensible girls, worried women, wanton women, and even a couple of garrulous grannies. *Grannies were getting younger, and younger these days*, she thought, wondering if the day would come when great-grandmothers would also need contraceptive advice.

She looked at her watch. 5:15 pm. Just one more patient to see, and then she could drive home and organise the children's tea. Hopefully, her husband would have remembered to call at the supermarket on his way home. If he hadn't he would get a flea in his ear.

She buzzed for her next patient.

Dr Julie, (she was known as Dr Julie to distinguish her from her husband, Dr Michael Smith), looked up from her notes as the door opened. A shadow of a woman entered the room and offered her a weary smile. She appeared to have lost all pride in her appearance. Her clothes were shabby and ill-fitting, her eyes tired, her face lined, her hair prematurely grey, and her hands, with their thick, calloused skin, spoke of long hours of hard work. She looked exhausted, and without waiting to be asked, sat down with a grateful sigh on the chair at the side of the doctor's desk.

'Am I glad to see you, Doctor.' It was a statement rather than a question. 'You know, I should have come years ago. Still better late than never, I suppose!' she continued.

'Is it Elsie Williams?' Dr Julie asked, glancing at her list of appointments.

'That's right, Elsie Williams of Rishworth Road, Bermondsey.'

She looked not a day less than forty, though her notes stated she was only 31.

Dr Julie liked to start the consultation with an open question, which allowed her an early insight into her patient's concerns and expectations.

'So what can I do for you?' she asked.

'I need to stop having any more babies!' Elsie said frankly.

'Well, that's what I'm here for,' Dr Julie replied, forcing her voice to sound more cheerful than she felt. 'How many children do you have?'

'Six.'

'Wow – you have been a busy girl, haven't you? And are they boys or girls?'

'They're all boys, and I really need to put a stop to it before I have a complete football team.'

'Boys are hard work. You must have your hands full, especially if you've got six of them.' Dr Julie responded, thinking how busy she was just having two little ones to cope with.

'And how old are they?

'My eldest is ten, and the latest arrival is just six months. And truly, with all the cleaning, washing, ironing, and cooking, I'm fair worn out, Doctor.'

'I'm sure you must be. And what have you called them all?'

'Dave.'

'And the others?'

'They're called Dave as well.'

There was a pause in the conversation while Dr Julie tried to digest this curious piece of information.

'But isn't that a bit confusing for them, all being called by the same name?'

'Not at all, Doctor. If they're arguing or fighting amongst themselves, as boys do, I just shout *'Dave – stop it'* and the trouble stops. Or, if I want to call them in for a meal, I shout *'Dave – tea's ready',* and they all come running. It works very well, and it's so simple.'

Dr Julie was puzzled. 'Yes, that's all very well, but suppose you just want to call one of them, say because he's got a dental appointment.'

'Well, Doctor, in that case, I just call him by his surname!'

My God, Dr Julie thought, this woman doesn't need contraception, she needs sterilisation!

A fast word about contraception; I asked a girl to go to bed with me and she said 'no'.

Woody Allen 1935

Life is a lottery

One summer's evening, the Lancashire police received reports that a car was being driven west at high speed, in poor visibility, on the east-bound carriageway of the M62 trans-Pennine motorway. They responded immediately, but before they were able to intercept the vehicle, it was involved in a head-on collision. Two people were killed. The police later reported that the driver of the car was driving under the influence of drugs and alcohol. At the time, there were hundreds of cars driving east on that stretch of road; families returning from a trip to the seaside, housewives going to the shops and commuters on their way home from work. But it wasn't any of them who died; it was Mary and Steven Baker, who were driving their three-year-old Fiat on their way to see their new-born grandson in Bradford. These two people were of course, completely innocent; it was simply their misfortune to be in the wrong place at the wrong time. Had they started their journey five minutes earlier or five minutes later, they would still be alive. Is what happened just bad luck or fate or, as some believe, preordained?

The same is true of knife crime. The heart and lungs are protected by the rib cage, the width of the ribs being equal in size to the space between them. When someone is stabbed in the chest, there is, therefore, a fifty-fifty chance that the knife will strike a rib. If it does, the result will be a small cut needing no more than a couple of skin stitches. No great harm is done, no time is lost off work and the incident may never come to the attention of the authorities. However, should the knife chance to slip between the ribs and penetrate the heart, the result may be sudden death, a murder charge, and a long period of imprisonment. The assailant, when striking the blow, has no idea what the result will be. In practice, he is putting himself and his victim, entirely in the hands of Lady Luck.

In practice, we have some control over how much we leave to luck. A cautious and sober individual will minimise risk, take precautions, and leave less to chance. Someone with a care-free attitude may take life as they find it, and allow luck to have a greater say in their destiny. Others may deliberately allow fate to determine their future. Should they be unable to make up their minds when a major decision has to be made, they may simply toss a coin to decide their course.

I've known a coin to be tossed to decide the future of others. On one occasion, when a medical appointment was being made, the selection committee could not agree which of two candidates to appoint. Both were suitable, and both had equal support amongst the panel. After hours of wrangling, with neither faction prepared to give ground, the decision was made by the flip of a fifty pence piece. One candidate was lucky, one unlucky. That coin determined which of them would get the job, which family would have to move house, and which of them would one day become an NHS consultant.

Most doctors and nurses will admit that luck has played a significant part in their careers. I certainly received no favours from Lady Luck on the day I took the exam which would determine whether I qualified as a doctor, instead, she smiled benignly on a fellow student friend of mine!

Having taken the written papers after five years at Medical School, we had to prove our competence in a clinical assessment at the bedside. It was a matter of chance which of several examiners would interrogate us, which patient we would examine, and what questions we would be asked.

My assessment started when I was given a sample of urine to test. We had been told that some of the samples contained blood, some sugar, others protein, and that some were normal. Mine tested positive for blood. So far, so good. I now had 15 minutes to wait before meeting my examiner. It seemed obvious that the initial questions would centre on the causes of blood in the urine, so I began to classify them in my mind.

There were the general abnormalities of blood clotting, such as haemophilia and anticoagulant therapy. Then there were local problems of the various parts of the waterworks system: diseases of the kidneys, such as stones and tumours, and abnormalities of the ureters, bladder, prostate, and urethra. Soon, I had the perfect answer organised in my mind. I was confident. I would dazzle the examiner, not just with my knowledge but with the structured way in which I presented the facts.

'Good morning, Sir,' I said when introduced to the examiner, a dour-looking Professor of Surgery from a neighbouring teaching hospital. I looked him straight in the eye, determined to impress.

'Have you examined the urine sample that you were given?' he asked.

'Yes, Sir, I have.'

'What did you find?'

'The presence of blood, Sir.'

'That's quite right. Not too difficult, I suppose, given that the urine was red!' His voice was quiet and held just a hint of sarcasm.

I was ready for him, my prepared answer on the tip of my tongue.

The examiner allowed a small, humourless smile to cross his face.

'Tell me, young man, about the causes of blood in the stool?'

In a confident voice, I began to answer.

'There are many causes of blood in the urine, Sir,' I said, 'and we can start by dividing them into general causes and local....'

'No,' he interrupted, the sarcasm now more pronounced than before. 'Didn't you hear what I said? I asked you tell me the causes of blood in the stool.'

'In the stool, Sir?'

'Yes, in the stool.' The voice was now mocking in tone. His bored expression had vanished, his smile now a satisfied beam.

What a bastard, I thought, wondering how often he had pulled this particular trick on other unsuspecting students.

Having prepared carefully a list of all the causes of blood in the urine, I was completely thrown to be asked for the causes of blood in the stool. My confidence evaporated, my mind became a blank.

I was angry with myself for making an assumption about the question I would be asked and furious with the examiner for the trick he had played on me. I became hot, I started to sweat, and still, my brain refused to function. *'Blood in the stool'*, he had said, *'blood in the stool'*. Slowly my mind cleared, but it was only after a good deal of prompting that I managed to stutter and stammer some sort of answer to the question. Inevitably, I received a very poor mark.

The experience of one of my fellow students, Graeme Boswell, was strikingly different. During his medical school days, he had spent part of his training on an Ear, Nose, and Throat unit. The consultant there was a pleasant, quietly-spoken, grey-haired, fifty-year-old called Miss Peterson. At the time, she was the only female surgeon in the hospital. One day, she was supervising while we students were examining each other's noses with a nasal speculum. Graeme had no difficulty looking up the nose of other students, but no-one was able to catch even a glimpse inside Graeme's nose. Miss Peterson came to see what the problem was.

She examined his nose and saw that it was blocked due to an old rugby injury.

'Can you breathe through that?' she asked.

'No,' was the reply. 'I can only breathe through my mouth, and everyone says I snore as well.'

'You need a sub-mucous resection,' Miss Peterson said, 'it's not a major operation. Go to my secretary and book a date. Tell her that I've said you can choose a date to fit in with your studies.'

Graeme duly had his surgery in the Easter vacation.

Twelve months later, who was Graeme lucky enough to meet in the medical examination, but Miss Peterson who immediately recognised him. She looked at his nose.

'Can you breathe through that?' she asked, not for the first time!

'No, I'm afraid I can't, and people still complain that I snore.'

She had a quick look at it. 'Hmm. I've not done a very good job there, have I? You need another operation. In the circumstances, I don't think I ought to ask you any questions. I'm certain you're going to pass this exam. Go and see my secretary, and book a date. Tell her that I've said you may pick a date before you take up your first job as a doctor.'

The next stage of the assessment was for Graeme to be observed whilst examining a patient. He feared the worst when he learned he was to meet the devious external examiner who had examined me and was known to have failed numerous candidates the previous year.

'Examine this patient's neck.' The instruction was curt, the voice severe.

Graeme looked at the patient's neck from the front and saw a goitre, a swelling of the thyroid gland. He was about to seek the patient's permission to palpate it when the examiner interrupted him.

'You have a cauliflower ear,' he exclaimed. 'How did you get that?'

'Lots of bumps and bruises, Sir. I did a bit of boxing and a lot of rugby!'

'And what's your name, young man?'

'Boswell, Sir, Graeme Boswell.'

'That rings a bell. Didn't you play for the United Provincial hospitals in the inter-hospital championships?'

'Yes, Sir.'

'Excellent, excellent! I used to play in those matches years ago, and I still enjoy going along to watch. It's good to see you again, Boswell. I've no further questions for you. You may go!'

So Graeme, lucky fellow, passed both assessments without being asked a single medical question.

'Lady Luck' is a fickle female. Should she smile upon you, you are truly blessed. Your journey through life will be smooth, and your dreams and ambitions will be fulfilled. But should 'Lady Luck' ignore you, or worse, frown upon you, then Heaven help you!

Thought for the day

In examinations, those who do not wish to know, ask questions of those who cannot tell.

Walter Raleigh 1861-1922

The Man with the Curious Limp

People say that in life, certain things are inevitable, meaning that, try as you may, you cannot avoid them; birth, for example, and death of course. For students and certainly for medical students, there is another inevitability: an examination in every subject at the end of every course. They also say that acceptance of what cannot be changed is the way to find peace and contentment. But how, I ask you, do you find this peace and contentment when faced with the trauma of these fearful examinations?

There are the hours spent swotting when you would much prefer to be socialising with your friends, or enjoying life in the countryside, or on the sports field. There are the sleepless nights as the day of the exam approaches, the worry as you try to anticipate what questions will be asked, and the conviction that your preparation is inadequate, and failure inevitable. Then the dreaded day arrives. You wake in the morning feeling nauseated, your palms are moist, and your bowels loose. With nerves on edge, you set out for the examination venue, arriving far too early. Then you assemble with your friends and fellow students outside the examination hall. The conversation is subdued, then dies away completely as you shuffle reluctantly into the building.

Inside the hall, the wooden desks and chairs are widely spaced in neat rows. The invigilator stands on the platform at the front and coughs to attract attention.

'The examination will last for three hours,' he says. 'In a moment, I shall walk around the hall and place the paper face down on the desk in front of you. You will not turn it over until I give the word. That is when your time begins.

There are four questions on the paper, and you must answer them all. Each question has equal weighting. You are therefore advised to spend an equal amount of time on each question. I will inform you when you have thirty minutes left. Is that clear to everyone?'

It's almost a relief when you finally see the paper, consider the questions, and begin to plan your answers. The first ten minutes pass slowly, then time gallops away. Surreptitiously, you look round and see that everyone else has their head down and is scribbling away furiously. *They will be doing far better than I am*, you say to yourself. You answer the easiest question first, spending more time on it than you should, then find when the thirty-minute bell rings, that you have yet to start the last question. In a panic, you end up sketching a skeleton of an answer, trying to include the most important points.

'Put your pens down now, please. Your time is up,' the invigilator calls, 'Stop writing, and turn your answers face down.'

You finish the sentence you are writing, hoping it may bring you that extra mark that will spell the difference between a pass and a fail, then reluctantly lay your pen to one side.

Immediately, conversations break out around the room. 'Silence please,' comes the order. 'There will be no talking until you have left the hall.'

Once outside, the candidates display a wide range of emotions, some strikingly confident, some cautiously satisfied, others visibly distressed. Everyone is talking at once, as the four questions are debated. Occasionally, you see a friend's face drop as you mention something they have forgotten. Far more frequently, as you listen, you realise others have remembered important facts that you have omitted.

I have my own painful memory of one occasion when the question concerned common conditions that may cause a child to walk with a limp. When in the examination hall, my mind had turned to all the conditions I'd read about in my orthopaedic textbook, as well as some I had seen in the orthopaedic ward: conditions such as congenital club foot, Perthes' disease, and Osgood-Schlatter's disease. I came away well-pleased with my answer, confident of getting a good mark. The moment I chatted with my friends, though, I was deflated.

'The commonest cause of a limp must be a stone in your shoe' said one.

'Or a 'dead leg' given by the bully in the school playground,' volunteered another.

'Or, perhaps an in-growing toenail, or maybe a twisted ankle playing football', said a third.

'And on a worldwide basis, probably TB of the knee,' was a further suggestion.

To my horror, I realised I'd not read the question properly. They hadn't asked for the medical causes of a limp, they'd asked for the *common* causes of a limp.

Immediately, my confidence collapsed, I hadn't mentioned any of these conditions, and I felt a complete fool. How often had I been told to read the question carefully, to answer the question as it was written, not as you think it ought to have been written? What an idiot I had been!

All this came to my mind recently when I was undergoing an ultra-sound examination to ascertain why my urinary stream was not as strong as it was when I was a young man and why I woke three times every night to have a pee. The radiologist was much the same age as I, well to be honest he was probably ten years younger, and as I was the last patient on his list, and we both had time on our hands, we ended up reminiscing about our medical careers. He told me a story of a patient with an unusual cause of a limp, a story that had been told to him by his medical father.

The story concerned a man who was seen walking past the windows of the hospital's orthopaedic department on a daily basis. He had a most peculiar gait. To describe his limp to you in words isn't easy, so I must ask you to try to visualise in your mind how he walked. He was hunched up and bending forward at the waist, with his arms in front of him, hands clenched together, level with his chest. Most peculiar of all, he was walking backward, not looking where he was going at all! Walking also appeared to be a great effort, for he was puffing and blowing like a steam engine. Unsurprisingly, he was progressing very slowly and seemed to be in a great deal of pain.

The junior nurses and doctors in the orthopaedic department were very puzzled and asked the consultant orthopaedic surgeon if he knew what the diagnosis was.

'Yes', he said, 'I do.'

'And....?'

'Well, it's probably best to go and ask him, because he knows what the problem is.'

So, the next day, when the man was passing, one of the nurses dashed out and asked him that very question. She returned a few minutes later, an amused look on her face.

'Well then, what's the diagnosis?' her friends demanded.

'You'll never guess,' she replied. 'He's pulling the Titanic safely back into port to stop her sinking.'

'He's doing what?'

'He's deluded. He wants to save the lives of the passengers on the Titanic. He's a patient at the Psychiatric Institute down the road.'

A Donation to Charity

'Hello Gerry, you don't mind me calling you Gerry, do you? Calling you Doctor would be a bit formal on a Saturday afternoon, wouldn't it, especially when you're out in the garden enjoying the sunshine. Obviously, I wouldn't dream of being so informal at the surgery, but we are neighbours after all, aren't we?'

Dr Parkinson was irritated, though far too polite to show it. His garden, especially his back garden, was his private reserve, somewhere where he liked to relax. Damn it. Surely he was entitled to unwind in peace and quiet after a hard week at the surgery.

'I've just popped round to see if you would mind sponsoring my Jimmy,' Annie Smithson continued. Apparently, her definition of 'neighbour' included anyone living within three streets of the doctor's house. 'He's going to run a kilometre with the cubs for charity.'

She turned to her son, who stood, hands in pockets, eyes glued to the ground, two steps behind her.

'Tell the nice Doctor what the money's for, Jimmy. Actually, he's a bit shy, so it will be best if I tell you. The scout hut needs a new roof, that's the one on the main road, not the one down the avenue next to the park. The roof leaks something terrible; they have to get buckets out to catch the drips every time it rains, so it's an excellent cause, don't you agree?'

Actually, her general practitioner didn't agree. Thanks to a lottery grant recently received, a new sports hall was being built only a stone's throw away. It would make an ideal venue for both of the scout groups. Annie, though, didn't give him a chance to say so. Scarcely pausing to take a breath, she continued.

'Actually, I'm glad I've bumped into you, especially as I've got Jimmy with me. He's developed a bit of a rash on his chest. He's not been ill with it, mind, well perhaps he's been a bit peaky, but they all get like that from time to time, don't they? Just pull up your shirt, Jimmy, and show the Doctor. Well, perhaps I'd better do it to save time. I know how busy you Doctors are and how your time is precious to you.'

Yes, my time is precious, Dr Parkinson thought, wondering how best to rid himself of this unwelcome visitor without appearing to be unacceptably rude or abrupt.

'There, can you see it. It's quite faint, isn't it, and it doesn't seem to hurt him. It doesn't hurt you, Jimmy, does it? No, of course, it doesn't, you'd have told me if it did, wouldn't you?

He's had all his ocular nations, Doctor, so it can't be anything serious. I wouldn't want you to think I'm one of those silly mums who think that vacillations cause all sorts of terrible diseases. Serves them right, though, doesn't it, if their kids get the measles if they ignore the doctor's advice.

Do you see it goes round the back a bit too? It only came on this morning. I suspect it must be something he's eaten. He went to a party yesterday at Molly Jones'; you know the posh lady who lives on The Grove, the one who's always telling you about her fancy holidays. She went to the Caribbean last winter, you know, on one of those fancy cruise liners. She insisted on telling me all about it. Blackpool's not good enough for the likes of her! It must have cost her a pretty packet. She's the one with all those funny food fads, 'faganism' I think it's called. Goodness knows what she gave the children to eat. Jimmy's used to the good, plain, wholesome food I give him, so I bet that's the cause of it. Anyway, it will probably be gone by tomorrow, so I'm not going to worry about it.

Oh, and while I'm here, Doctor, would you cast your eye on this little lump on my arm. It'll save me going to the surgery. It can take two or three weeks to get an appointment these days, can't it – but I guess you know that already! In the old days, before they had appointments, you just turned up, and the doctor saw everyone who came. That was much better. Mind you, you often had to wait an hour or more to be seen. Swings and roundabouts, I guess.

There, can you see it? It's very small, I grant you, and it really causes me no trouble, but I just want you to tell me it's nothing serious. It's the same colour as the rest of my skin, not like those malign ova things that you read about. You really can't be too careful with lumps, can you? All of poor Mrs Crabshaw's troubles started with a little lump, didn't they, and just look at her now. She in the hospice, isn't she, and we all know where that will end. I don't think my lump is the result of an injury or anything. I don't remember knocking it at all. I suppose it will go away on its own, but I'm pleased if you don't think it's anything to worry about.

The Hospice is a very worthwhile charity, of course, but it doesn't help the local youngsters, does it, whereas scouting gives them something to do, something to keep them out of mischief.

They always say the devil find's work for idle hands don't they?

Oh, is that a ten-pound note, that's so kind of you, Doctor. Jimmy say, 'Thank you' to the nice Doctor. He really is grateful, Doctor, though he doesn't say a lot, he's just a bit shy. That will help the Scout Hut Roof Fund a great deal. Very generous of you, I'm sure.

Well, I must be running along now, I've got a few jobs to do in my own garden, so I've no time to waste.

Thank you, Doctor. You've been so kind and you've really put my mind at rest. I shall sleep so much better tonight.

Say goodbye to the Doctor, Jimmy; there's a good boy.'

Dr Parkinson watched her as she left, little Jimmy trailing behind her. He sighed, put his wallet back in his trouser pocket, and turned back to continue pruning his roses. His visitors were disappearing around the side of the house when he heard Jimmy's voice for the first time.

'Can I have that ice cream now, Mum?

'Yes, you can – but the rest is for my ciggies.'

An Anglo German Misunderstanding

Hans Schmidt had lived all his life in the village of Tutzing, on the shores of Lake Starnberg, in Southern Germany. At the age of 21, he had married his childhood sweetheart, Gerda, and opened a small bakery, supplying bread and cakes to the local community. When his working days were over, the couple remained in Tutzing amongst their long-standing friends and acquaintances. Hans was happy to keep a few hens and grow his own vegetables; Gerda was content to knit, sew, and to tend the flowers in their local church.

Then the first of two disasters struck: Hans collapsed and died from a massive heart attack. It came without warning one late summer's afternoon, whilst he was hoeing the weeds in the garden. Gerda was devastated. Hans had always been there for her; he had run the family finances, maintained the house, garden, and car, and organised their occasional holidays. Essentially, he had been her rock, making all the decisions, but in protecting her from all responsibility, he had left her ill prepared to live life on her own, as a widow.

Gerda was now 82-years-old, alone, and quite unable to cope. Fortunately however, they had a son called Helmut who, after obtaining a language degree at the University in Munich, had found employment in the German Embassy in London. He had married an English girl, and settled in Camberwell, south of the river. Helmut, seeing that his mother was struggling, invited her to come for an extended stay, as a trial to see if a permanent move to England would be in Gerda's best interests.

It was then that the second disaster occurred. Gerda had a stroke and was admitted to the hospital. The stroke paralysed her right arm and right leg, indicating that the damage was to the left side of her brain. She was also unable to communicate and the doctors needed to understand the reason for this. There were two possibilities. The first was expressive aphasia, a condition in which, although unable to produce speech, she could understand what was being said to her. The second possibility was receptive aphasia; when the brain damage has rendered her unable to understand the meaning of words spoken to her.

It was important for the doctors to understand the nature of the aphasia from which she was suffering, partly because it would tell them which area of the brain was affected, but mainly so that the speech therapists would know the best way to help her. The doctor's difficulties in making the distinction were, of course, compounded because Gerda did not speak any English.

The junior doctor on the Care of the Elderly female ward was Rob Martin, who spoke a little French but whose German was limited to the words *'zwei bier bitte'*, (two biers please) learned when, many years previously, he had been on a school skiing trip to the Austrian Alps. Distinguishing between expressive and receptive aphasia in a non-English speaking German national was way beyond him, but he had a trick up his sleeve. It happened that the junior doctor on the male ward at this time was Hans Meyer, who had moved with his parents to England when he was a boy and who had studied medicine at Sheffield University. Hans was a delightful character with a good sense of humour.

'I am a geriatric doctor,' he used to say to his English friends. 'Do you know what a geriatric is? He's a German centre-forward who scores a hat trick against England and knocks them out of the World Cup.'

'Hans,' Rob said to his colleague, 'have you five minutes to help me with a little problem?'

He went on to describe Gerda's speech problem and the need to distinguish between the two types of aphasia.

Hans was only too pleased to help, so together they went to Gerda's bedside. The way to resolve the riddle was to discover whether Gerda could follow simple instruction.

'Close your eyes,' Hans instructed.

There was no response at all from Gerda, and it appeared she was oblivious to the spoken word.

'Try again,' Rob said.

'I want you to close your eyes, Gerda,' Hans repeated a little louder.

There was still no response.

Hans put his mouth close to Gerda's ear.

'CLOSE YOUR EYES!' he shouted.

Rob fell about laughing. 'She's German, Hans,' he said, 'and so are you. Try speaking in German.'

'Schliebedeine augen,' Hans said to Gerda when he had recovered from his embarrassment – and she did!

If you understand English, press one,
If you don't understand English, press two.

Anonymous

A box of Crystalline Fruits

The President of the Royal Society of London, the world's oldest independent scientific academy, suffered from haemorrhoids. He had put up with their itching, discomfort, and occasional bleeding for many years, partly because he was reluctant to take time off work, but mainly because the prospect of an operation and an anaesthetic frightened him. The pain was at its most severe when he sat through the many Society dinners that were a major part of the President's life. Eventually, however, the time came when even the finest French clarets and purest Scottish malt whiskies provided no relief, and he was forced to face his fears and seek relief.

He sought advice from the Chairman of the British Medical Association, a recently-retired professor, who happened to be a surgeon. The Royal Society President clearly failed to appreciate that any surgeon who has risen to such an exalted position has inevitably spent the bulk of his or her career doing research and committee work and throughout his career would have delegated humble haemorrhoid operations to their trainees. The President would have been far wiser to consult a jobbing surgeon in a District General Hospital who operates on piles several times each week.

The BMA Chairman, however, was not unaware of his own limitations and, following the lead taken by the 78 year old 'Royal Obstetrician' who had the dubious honour, but major responsibility, of delivering the many royal babies that the monarchy produce these days, was wise enough to arrange for a very experienced trainee, and a senior theatre sister to be present when the surgery was undertaken. Their role was to hold his hand, to ensure that things went well, and to take the flack if they didn't.

Fortunately, perhaps surprisingly, the operation proceeded smoothly, and the Royal Society President's generously-proportioned rear was relieved of the painful, bleeding piles that had caused him to wriggle and squirm through so many long and tedious committee meetings. Equally fortuitously, his convalescence was uncomplicated, and within a month, he was back at work. Having suffered from the inconvenience and discomfort of his haemorrhoids for many years, he was naturally extremely grateful to the BMA chairman and effusive with his thanks.

Some months later, when he had long since forgotten performing the surgery, (his memory declining in tandem with his advancing age), the BMA Chairman received a telephone call from the President's secretary inviting him to be an honoured guest at the grand dinner which concluded the Royal Society's annual conference. It was to be held during the third week in December. The secretary made it clear that he would not be required to speak; the invitation was simply the President's way of expressing his personal gratitude for the service he had rendered.

'Oh, you mean that little job I undertook for the President,' he said.

'Yes, that's right,' the secretary replied, 'but also of course, for your lifelong commitment to medicine. I've also been requested to ask what special item you would like to receive as a Christmas present.'

Modestly, he tried to decline, saying he'd been pleased to have been able to help and that a present really wasn't necessary. But the secretary was insistent. He thought quickly. Thanks to representing the BMA abroad on many occasions, he already had a cupboard full of gifts, mostly symbolic, and of little practical use, his drinks cabinet was well stocked with whisky and gin, so he simply said that a small box of crystalline fruits would be appreciated.

***

The theme of the Christmas Conference was 'Making a Difference in the World'. It had gone well. Delegates from many countries had attended and contributed to its success. Favourable reports had already appeared in the international press. The BMA Chairman thoroughly enjoyed the gourmet dinner which followed the closing ceremony. He felt privileged to be sitting at the top table in affable company, whilst good quality wines flowed freely. In a mellow mood, puffing his cigar and with a whisky to hand, he sat back in his chair as the President rose to close the conference with a few well-chosen final words.

As is always the case, much of what he said could have been predicted. He thanked all those who had contributed papers and those who had sponsored the event. He praised the Society's staff for organising the meeting and announced the date and theme for the next annual conference.

Then turning to the notes he held in his hand, he came to his concluding remarks.

'The Royal Society is fortunate enough to hear the views and ambitions of many of the world's most influential people, and we have asked some of them the single thing they would most like for Christmas. The President of the Royal College of Physicians said the elimination of all infectious diseases, the Chairman of UNICEF said clean, drinking water for all children worldwide and the Chairman of the British Medical Association said.........a small box of crystalline fruits.'

Unfit for Human Consumption

'Telephone for you, Mr Gregg.'

The consultant groaned, annoyed that people rang in the middle of a Monday morning clinic, interrupting him when he was busy with patients.

'Is it urgent?' he asked of the nurse who had brought the message.

Apparently, it was, so he apologised to the 'dishabille' patient.

The caller was not known to Mr Gregg but introduced himself as Dr Crispen Brown, an occupational health doctor who also acted as consultant to various local manufacturers, including the giant British Bread Baking Company (BBBC) who had a large factory only a mile from the hospital. Their bread, biscuits, and cakes were a household name throughout the country, as was their advertising slogan 'The BBBC – better than the BBC – our bread makes great news'.

'I'm afraid we have an urgent problem at the factory,' Dr Brown explained. 'An unfortunate incident occurred this morning, and I need your advice as to whether a certain batch of loaves is fit to be sold.'

'What precisely is the problem?' Mr Gregg asked.

'I'd rather not say any more on the phone if you don't mind; it's rather sensitive. I wouldn't want any word of this to reach public ears. Would you mind if we met privately somewhere?'

'OK. Meet me at the hospital at, say 5.30. I should be through by then.'

'No, I should prefer to meet you at home, either yours or mine, I don't mind.'

Mr Gregg suggested the following weekend, but this apparently wasn't soon enough, so reluctantly, he agreed that Dr Crispen Brown could come to his home that evening. He didn't like intrusions into his private life, but it seemed preferable to finding his way to Dr Brown's house.

As he replaced the phone, he was irritated. His arm had been twisted such that he'd ended up inviting a stranger to his home, without the slightest idea of the reason, though he was undeniably curious as to the nature of the problem. He only hoped it was a matter of some significance and not a wild goose chase.

Crispen Brown proved to be a slightly-built man, aged about fifty, grey in appearance and timid of manner. He had a pallid complexion, grey hair, a grey suit which showed signs of wear at the elbows and cuffs, and he spoke hesitantly in a voice that was scarcely more than a whisper.

'I'm so sorry to barge in on you in this manner,' he began, 'but there's been an unfortunate incident at the factory. Regrettably, some foreign bodies have been incorporated into a batch of loaves we've baked. I would be so grateful if you would advise whether the bread is fit to be sold and eaten.'

He went on to explain in meticulous and time-consuming detail that each Sunday night, the bread production line stopped to allow the various industrial machines to be 'deep cleaned'. This included the commercial 'mixer', a machine very similar to a domestic food mixer but very much larger; the bowl was about ten feet across and ten feet deep.

A man was lowered into the bowl to clean it, using a large 'paddle', a piece of wood shaped like an oar, to scrape the bowl before it was 'power-hosed' clean. Carelessly, the worker had left the paddle in the bowl where it had remained until the next morning, when flour, yeast, salt, and water were added, and the giant mixer switched on. The result was that the wooden paddle was smashed, then splintered into a thousand pieces. The dough had been moulded, baked, and then divided into loaves before being sliced and packaged. Fortunately, the mistake was spotted by the quality control department before the resulting loaves left the factory.

Mr Gregg listened somewhat impatiently as Dr Brown related this story. At 7 pm on a Monday evening, having put in a long day at the hospital, he would normally already have enjoyed his pre-prandial drink and be sitting around the table with his wife tucking into his dinner. It seemed to him that this long preamble was unnecessary. All Dr Brown needed to do was to show him a sample of the bread. Eventually, he did so, producing from his bag a small white loaf. Rather dramatically, he then produced a breadboard and a sharp knife.

The knife cut through the loaf with difficulty, revealing the splinters of wood. Some were a couple of inches long and as sharp as a needle at both ends.

'It's blatantly obvious no-one could eat those,' Mr Gregg exclaimed, 'their guts would be cut to shreds. It wouldn't be safe to feed them to elephants! Anyone can see that. Why on earth have you bothered to come all this way for me to confirm what you must surely already know?'

Crispen Brown had the grace to look apologetic.

'Yes, I do know,' he whispered, 'and I'm sorry it's been necessary to trouble you. But to discard the whole of a morning's production will cost the company in excess of fifty thousand pounds. I'm required to get a second opinion to confirm my view.

You will, of course, be compensated for your time,' he added swiftly, obviously realising that Mr Gregg was not best pleased to be giving up his time to offer medical advice that his five-year-old son could have given.

And indeed, he was rewarded. He thought perhaps he might be given a year's supply of biscuits and cakes, but no, within the week, a letter of thanks arrived together with a cheque that was more valuable to him than a whole day's work at the hospital.

Thought for the day

England is the only country in the world where the food is more dangerous than sex.

Jackie Mason 1931

James Bond

Ian was a general practitioner in Herefordshire and enjoyed his life there immensely. He found that one of the delights of being a doctor in a rural practice was that he was able to blend seamlessly into country life although, like the local vicar, publican, and vet, he was distinguished by virtue of his profession. Living within his practice area, buying groceries at the village shop, and drinking in the village pub, he rubbed shoulders with his patients every day and built a solid relationship with them. He didn't mind too much if they sought his advice out of hours when one of their children developed a rash or cut their leg and, in return, there was always someone to lend a hand with some heavy job in the garden, or if a baby sitter was needed at short notice.

There were also country pursuits to be enjoyed, riding being Ian's favourite pastime. He had a couple of horses stabled at his home and a three-acre paddock in which they could graze. He also enjoyed country dances, and on this beautiful, late summer's evening, he and his wife, Carol, were getting dressed to attend one of the highlights of the village calendar, the annual charity dinner-dance which was held at the Community Hall. This year's chosen charity was the local Hospice.

Ian looked at himself in the mirror; black dinner jacket, frilly white shirt, black bow tie, and shiny black shoes. Very smart, not bad for a man of 50, he said to himself.

Carol came over, straightened his tie a fraction, and brushed some non-existent speck from the shoulder of his jacket.

'You do scrub up quite well when you make an effort,' she said affectionately as she gave him a kiss on the cheek.

Ian was glancing in the mirror again to check for any trace of lipstick on his cheek when there was a loud banging on the front door.

'Oh, no, 'Carol said, 'surely you're not going to get called out now.'

Ian went downstairs to find a policeman standing on the front doorstep.

The constable looked at Ian's attire in some surprise

'Sorry to trouble you, Doctor, especially as it looks as if you're about to go out, but I'm afraid I need your help. A young girl has fallen off a horse down by the river, she seems to have concussion, and may have a broken leg. Her friend rode up to the road and flagged me down.'

Ian feared the worst, as these were undoubtedly two young teenage girls from the village, daughters of a friend of his, who had taken his two horses out for a summer evening ride. He just hoped the injured girl had been wearing a riding helmet. One of the young men from the village had recently come off his horse and, not wearing a helmet, had suffered some slight but permanent brain damage.

'Right,' Ian said to the policeman, 'I'll come at once.'

Resplendent in his evening dress and shiny shoes, Ian was whisked in the police car, siren blaring, to the end of the track, where one of the girls was anxiously waiting holding the two horses.

To the policeman's great surprise, Ian swiftly mounted one of the horses and galloped down the track and across the field to the river.

He found the other girl lying in the grass next to the track on a sharp bend. Apparently the two friends had been racing, and, when they got to the bend, her horse had slipped and fallen on its side, throwing its young rider to the ground.

Ian arrived at full gallop, then went into four-hoofed-braking mode, bringing up an impressive cloud of dust. He leapt off the horse, brushed the dust off his jacket, adjusted his bow tie and strode up to attend to the young lady.

Expecting effusive thanks, he was a more than a little disappointed when she said, 'Oh, I thought James Bond had come to rescue me, but it's only you!'

What a blow to Ian's ego!

She didn't have a concussion, merely a couple of fractured metatarsals where her foot had been trapped in the stirrups.

Kitty

On a Saturday evening Mabel, a quiet retiring spinster, was invariably to be found at home, sitting in her favourite armchair, her knitting needles hard at work, and her curtains tightly drawn. Her only companions were Kitty, her cat, and the comforting background chatter of the radio. With midnight approaching on this particular Saturday, however, she was not at home; she was in the waiting room of the casualty department of her local hospital.

Only rarely did Mabel leave the security of her home, and then only to slip to the shops or to worship at her local church on a Sunday morning. She declined invitations to join the Women's Institute or to participate in church social activities. Not that she had always been like this. As a schoolgirl and in her late teens and early twenties, she had been a lively, outgoing and popular individual. Never short of friends, she had enjoyed dances and trips to the cinema and had generally been the life and soul of any party.

The event that caused this transformation occurred in 1914, when Charlie, the young man to whom she was engaged, enlisted in the Manchester Pals; part of Lord Kitchener's New Army. Charlie had travelled to France and became one of the thousands who lost their lives at the Battle of the Somme. The light went out of Mabel's life, and from that day to this, she carried his memory in her heart and his photograph in the handbag that was always at her side.

Whilst waiting to be seen, she had heard language and witnessed events that were entirely foreign to her, reinforcing her belief that her sheltered life suited her well. Several times, experiencing a rising sense of panic, she felt an urge to leave the hospital and return to the sanctuary of her own home, but on each occasion, she resisted. She needed medical advice, so she forced herself to wait. She just wished that the wait would soon be over. She tried to calm herself by taking slow, deep breaths. She distracted herself by studying the tired, tatty posters on the equally tired and tatty walls. *'Protect yourself – use a sheath,'* she read alongside a graphic depiction of the male anatomy. *'She may look clean but syphilis and gonorrhoea can kill,'* she read on another, illustrated by a tart chatting to a sailor. She averted her gaze in disgust.

Over an hour later, to her enormous relief, she heard her name called over the tannoy; *'Mabel Mullins to cubicle three please.'*

Steve, the Casualty Officer, emptied the cubicles in order; cubicle one, cubicle two, cubicle three. Then back to cubicle one. It may be imagined that it was boring, but it wasn't. Each cubicle held a new patient, a different problem, and a fresh challenge. Already that day, he had removed a peanut from the nose of a three-year-old girl. Her elder brother had placed it there in a vain attempt to control her fit of sneezing! He had treated a builder who had dropped a lump hammer on his foot. Foolishly, he had left his steel-capped boots at home and gone to work wearing open-toed sandals! Later, there had been a housewife who had cut her hand whilst filleting fish, an office worker with indigestion, and an elderly man with concussion sustained in a road traffic accident. It had been a typical shift in a busy casualty department. Fortunately, none of the patients had been seriously injured, and Steve had managed to treat them all without calling for senior advice.

It was now two in the morning, and he was sitting in the office, sharing a well-earned pot of tea and some hot buttered toast with the nursing sister. The staff nurse popped her head around the door. She had a huge grin on her face.

'I've just put a patient into cubicle three,' she said above the background noise. 'She's says she's got abdominal pain.'

The drunk whose head wound had just been stitched was groaning as he stumbled towards the exit, assisted by one of the night porters. A young woman, who had swallowed a handful of sleeping tablets in a futile attempt to convince her boyfriend of her undying love, was sobbing gently in an adjacent cubicle. She hadn't enjoyed having her stomach pumped out. Steve was weary. It had been a long day. He'd been hoping no more patients would require his attention, and that he would be able to snatch a couple of hours sleep before morning. He saw nothing remotely amusing about having to attend yet another patient.

'And what's so funny about that?' he asked.

'You'll find out when you see her.'

'Is it urgent, or can I finish my tea?'

'I really don't know.' The staff nurse was laughing. 'It's difficult to say.'

It was clear there was something about the patient in cubicle three that she found highly entertaining. It didn't sound as if the problem was sufficiently urgent for Steve to interrupt his snack, but curiosity got the better of him. He went to discover what it was that the staff nurse found so amusing.

Patients from all walks of life attended a hospital's accident department; injuries and illness having no respect for social class or status, but when Steve saw this particular lady, she looked distinctly out of place. She was stoutly built and was sitting primly to attention; knees and ankles clamped tightly together. On her head she wore what appeared to be a knitted woollen tea cosy, decorated with a bold and colourful floral design. A large string of multi-coloured glass beads hung around her neck over her cardigan, again hand-knitted, the colours and design matching her hat. A heavy tweed skirt, a pair of thick woollen socks and leather walking boots completed her outfit. With her round, gentle face and grey hair, matching whiskers on upper lip and chin, she reminded Steve of the maiden aunt who visited his family home each Christmas when he was a child. Her hugs and kisses were only tolerated because they were followed by the gift of a crisp five pound note which his father promptly confiscated *'for safe-keeping'.*

On her lap, Miss Mullins held a wicker basket covered with a tea towel. Steve thought she would have looked more at home attending a village craft fair on a Saturday afternoon, than a city centre casualty department in the small hours of Sunday morning. She didn't appear to be in any pain or distress; indeed, she looked sheepish rather than ill.

Steve introduced himself, sounding irritated. His first impression was that this lady had no need to attend casualty or to waste time which he would have preferred to spend tucked up in a nice warm bed.

'Hello, I'm Dr Williams. I believe you have tummy ache.'

Miss Mullins looked embarrassed and sounded apologetic.

'No,' she said, 'actually I haven't, though I confess that's what I told the lady at the reception desk. If she'd known what I really wanted, she wouldn't have allowed me in. And I do so desperately need to see you. The truth is there's nothing the matter with me. It's Kitty.'

Gently she took the tea towel from the basket and revealed a large, but distinctly unhappy-looking cat, which was lying on a pad of heavily blood-stained cotton wool. The cat mewed in a weak and pitiful way as she stroked it lovingly.

'Look,' Steve said defensively, 'I'm not a vet. I don't know anything about cats.'

'I know you're not a vet,' she said softly, 'but you've studied medicine; you must have some ideas.'

Her concern for her cat was clearly genuine, and she was obviously desperate for some assistance. Steve was tempted to end the consultation there and then, rather than make any further enquiries. He was aware that the more involved he became, the more difficult it would be for him to extricate himself from the situation. There were a bed and the prospect of sleep waiting for him when the cubicles had been cleared. He wasn't paid to look after cats; his responsibility was to care for humans, not animals. It was, however, the look in her eyes, begging for help that made him weaken.

'What do you think is the matter with it?'

'Not *'it'*, Doctor. Kitty is female, and I think she must be pregnant. I know I should have taken her to the vet long ago to get her doctored, but I couldn't bear to think of Kitty having an operation. I thought that if I kept a close eye on her, this wouldn't happen.'

Knowing how cats love to wander the lonely streets and dark gardens at night, Steve considered this to be highly optimistic.

'And what makes you think she might be pregnant?'

'Well, she has been trying to make a nest in the backroom and has been 'yowling' something terrible. It's been so bad that I've had complaints from the neighbours. And now Kitty is in a lot of pain. I suspect she's in labour, and I can't bear to see her suffer.'

Tears filled her eyes as she lifted the large tabby out of the basket, placed the basket on the floor, then sat with the cat on her knee, gently stroking the fur on the back of its neck, and making soft cooing sounds.

'Look,' Steve said desperately, still looking for an early exit strategy, 'I really don't know anything about cats. When I was a lad at home, I had a couple of white mice, a stick insect, and a budgerigar. And there was a time when my father kept chickens in the back garden, but we never had a cat or a dog.'

With tears now rolling down her cheeks, Miss Mullins reached for Steve's hand and pleaded. 'But you will look at her for me, won't you, Doctor? She's so weak and lethargic now, and she's lost such a lot of blood. I'm afraid she's going to die.'

It was a request that was impossible to refuse, so crouching down beside her; Steve took the cat in his arms. It failed to react in any way to being handled by a stranger. It just lay, with eyes glazed, its head lolling weakly from side to side. The cat's abdomen was swollen, which suggested that it could be pregnant, and from time to time, its whole body went rigid and quivered as if it was experiencing a spasm of pain. Also, despite having no knowledge of feline anatomy, Steve could see that Kitty was bleeding from an orifice that he assumed to be the vagina.

Steve recognised that he was out of his depth; this was a situation he was unable to resolve on his own. Despite having treated thirty or more human patients during the course of the day without recourse to assistance, he needed help with this veterinary case. However, he certainly couldn't ring his boss, to whom he would normally turn for guidance on a diagnostic problem. Disturbing a consultant surgeon in the middle of the night to seek advice on a sick cat would torpedo all chance of future promotion – he would probably end his days as a lonely general practitioner on some far-flung Scottish island. Hoping that, by chance, there might be someone in the department who knew more about pregnant cats than he did, he lifted Kitty back into her basket, covered her with the tea towel and then asked Miss Mullins to accompany him to the office.

Bill Makin, the medical registrar, was there, together with the casualty sister. They were chatting with a couple of ambulance men, who were enjoying a break, whilst waiting for their next call.

'Does anybody know anything about pregnant cats?' Steve asked as he ushered Miss Mullins through the door. The question was something of a 'conversation stopper' but immediately George, one of the ambulance drivers, a rotund, ruddy-faced man in his fifties, expressed interest.

'Yes, I do. I've kept cats for years. Indeed, I breed them. It is a hobby of mine.'

'Excellent,' Steve replied, much relieved, 'because I've got a rather unhappy moggy here that seems to be struggling in labour.'

Quickly, George took a concise clinical history from Miss Mullins that would have done credit to any medical practitioner. He ascertained that in the last few days, as well as 'yowling' and attempting to create a nest, Kitty had lost interest in food, had been anxious and restless, and had spent many hours licking her belly and perineum.

He carefully examined the cat's abdomen and confirmed that she was indeed in labour. Then he voiced concern that the labour had lasted significantly longer than the three hours that was normal for a cat, adding that the bleeding was much heavier than he had previously witnessed. He obviously shared Miss Mullins' anxiety about the matter.

'For some reason, the kittens aren't coming through as they should,' he said. 'There must be a blockage of some sort. I really think this cat ought to be seen by a vet.'

'Or by an obstetrician,' Bill Makin remarked. 'I've already been on the telephone to St Margaret's Maternity Hospital earlier this evening about one of our cases. My old pal, David Winterbourne, is on duty there tonight. He and I were students together. We'll send Kitty there. He's sure to know what to do. I'll give him a ring.'

It was the nursing sister who spotted the obvious flaw in this plan.

'You really can't send a cat to a maternity hospital, even if she is pregnant,' she protested.

'Of course, I can,' replied the registrar cheerfully. 'I've known David for years, he won't mind in the least.'

'And we can run her there,' said George, knowing that St Margaret's was only half a mile away. 'We're not doing anything at the moment; just sitting here twiddling our thumbs.'

Bill Makin reached for the phone and rang his friend. The casualty staff, of course, were only able to hear one end of the conversation.

'I'm sorry to trouble you twice in one evening, David,' he said, 'but I'm afraid I need advice on another patient. It's a first pregnancy and a bit complex. As you know, I'm no expert in obstetrical matters, but I have a sneaking suspicion that this may be multiple pregnancies. She's in labour; probably has been for four or five hours now, and she's started to bleed quite heavily. She's in a lot of pain too and doesn't look at all well. I'd be grateful if you would take a look at her.'

There was a pause, but those listening in the office could imagine what was being said at the other end of the line, even though they couldn't hear it.

'No, she's not one of your patients.'

Another pause.

'I'm afraid she's had no antenatal care whatsoever. This is the first time anybody has realised that she's pregnant. I think she's been a little secretive about it.'

There was a longer pause. 'Yes, I know. Some people blame the schools, others blame the government, but personally, I think poor parenting has a lot to do with it, and there's no shortage of contraceptive advice available these days, is there? Mind you, I don't think she's the brightest of God's creatures. Maybe she's the sort that just can't say no.'

Another pause, shorter this time.

'No, I haven't remonstrated with her; I'll leave that to you. But I think I should warn you, she's a bit woolly-headed. I very much doubt that she'll understand. Her mother is with her, though,' he said, glancing at Miss Mullins. 'She seems quite sensible and may be able to keep an eye on things in the future.'

Another pause.

'Look, David, I'm a chest physician. Anything below the belt is a 'no-go' area for me. In my speciality, we don't go delving or diving into deep, dark holes. I wouldn't know where to find the cervix, let alone say whether it was dilated.'

Another pause.

'OK, and thanks for agreeing to see her. She's called Kitty by the way. I'm not sure what her surname is. She'll be coming by ambulance, and I'll have her with you within twenty minutes. Thanks David. It's very good of you.'

Bill smiled as he continued to listen.

'Yes, fair enough. I owe you one. I'll buy you a drink next time we meet. Goodnight, and thanks again.' Then as an afterthought, he added, 'Oh, and David, perhaps you would let me know how things turn out.'

He turned to face the group who had been listening intently to the telephone conversation. They all realised he'd failed to inform his friend that the patient was a cat.

'David says he's sick and tired of silly young girls who get themselves pregnant, and then are so ashamed that they hide themselves away, thinking they can cope all on their own, but who then turn up in labour having had no antenatal care at all. When he's sorted Kitty out, he intends to give her a firm lecture on the facts of life.'

He turned to the ambulance men.

'Are you sure you're able to take Kitty to St Margaret's? I wouldn't want you to get into any trouble.'

'Of course, we're sure,' said George. 'Nobody at Ambulance Control is going to know anything about it, because it's not going to get recorded in our log. We'll have her there in two ticks.'

George picked up Kitty and the basket, his colleague took Miss Mullins by the arm, and they started towards the door.

Miss Mullins turned a grateful smile on her face. 'Thank you all so much. You really have been most kind.'

'It's been a joint effort,' David replied, 'and our pleasure. I hope all turns out well.'

***

Work in the casualty department continued, but two hours later, Miss Mullins was back, cradling her basket in her arms with great care. She had made the return journey from St Margaret's, albeit this time on foot. She looked overjoyed, beaming from ear to ear, bursting to tell what had happened.

'I just had to let you see,' she said.

Gently, she placed the basket on a chair, then lifted a corner of the towel and showed everyone her beloved cat. Kitty was now lying contentedly in the basket, tenderly licking three tiny balls of fur that were snuggled up to her belly, their eyes closed. She handed Sister a letter.

'This is from the doctor at St Margaret's. He was just as kind as you were.'

Sister opened the envelope.

'*Dear Casualty Staff,*' it read. '*You were quite right. This was indeed multiple pregnancies; triplets in fact. But all has turned out well. As you see, mother and babies are all fine despite the lack of antenatal care. To avoid further problems, I have taken the liberty of giving Kitty's 'mother' some contraceptive advice.*

Kind regards,
David

'What's That You Said, Doctor?'

In these days of political correctness, one has to be careful not to cross the line of propriety; that is always assuming you know where that line is! In years gone by, it was possible to tell jokes about other countries or religions with impunity. The English could joke about the Irish, the French could poke fun at the Belgians, and the Austrians could enjoy a laugh at the expense of the Germans; but not so today. The exception appears to be if one tells a joke about oneself or one's own kind. It seems that a Scot is able to tell a joke which hints at the miserly reputation of his compatriots, which would not be acceptable if told by an Englishman. Take this example....

Jock turns to his wife, as he is about to go to the pub, and says 'Put your winter coat and hat on, Luv.'
'That's nice,' she replies, 'are you taking me out tonight?'
'No lass, not tonight.'
'Well then, why do I need to put my coat on?'
'I'm turning the central heating off while I'm out.' Jock replies.

Now I ask you, would that be acceptable if told by an Englishman?

With that in mind, here is a tale in which misunderstandings result from a patient's deafness. I claim impunity from criticism because I wear a pair of hearing aids myself!

Mr Bentley, the surgeon, was introduced by his junior staff to an elderly spinster called Esme Morris. Unfortunately, she had developed a tumour on her bowel and had been admitted to have a length of her colon removed. Esme was not only elderly, but also very frail and chesty.

To ensure she was fully aware of the potential benefits and complications of the proposed surgery, the consultant embarked on a detailed explanation of her operation but struggled because of Esme's profound deafness. The cotton screens were pulled around the bed, which provided visual privacy but, of course, didn't prevent conversations being overheard, particularly since the dialogue was conducted in loud voices. The surgeon was particularly keen to stress to his patient the importance of early physiotherapy and ambulation after her operation. There was good reason for this, the incidence of chest infections and blood clots in the legs being much reduced if patients mobilize quickly. Mr Bentley tapped Esme's legs.

'I want you to get these legs of yours moving after your operation.'

'What's that you say, Doctor?'

'I said exercise your legs after your operation,' he shouted tapping her legs again.

'Yes, Doctor, if you say so.'

He got hold of Esme's hands and waved them vigorously in the air. 'And get these arms moving as well.'

'Say that again, Doctor. I can't hear you?'

Again the surgeon shouted back. 'I want you to get these arms of yours moving after your operation.'

'Yes, Doctor, I will.'

'And I want you to take some nice big breaths.'

'You'll have to speak louder, Doctor.'

Mr Bentley's voice boomed across the ward, as he tapped Esme's chest.

'Nice big breaths.'

Esme cackled back at him, her voice shrill and penetrating, 'I'm not as big as I used to be, Doctor. All the boys used to say I was a big, bonny girl in the old days. But I'm surprised at you, being a doctor and saying such a thing.'

The surgeon, a gentlemanly bachelor, blushed to the roots of his silver hair and there were gales of laughter from the unseen audience behind the screens.

***

When Mr Bentley saw Esme after her surgery, his conversation with her again provided amusement, not only for the doctors and nurses who accompanied him but also for the patients in the vicinity.

Esme had successfully negotiated her operation, and the consultant wanted to know whether her bowels were returning to normal.

'Have you passed any flatus yet?' he asked.

'What's that you say, Doctor? You'll have to speak up a bit.'

'Have you passed any flatus?'

'Sorry, I still can't hear you,' replied Esme. 'I'm a bit deaf, you know.'

'Have you passed any wind yet?' he responded even louder than before.

'I still can't hear you, Doctor.'

'Have you farted?' Mr Bentley roared at the top of his voice.

Esme laughed and shouted back, 'No, Doctor, it must be one of you.'

Thought for the day

The most happy marriage I can picture or imagine would be the union of a deaf man to a blind woman.

Samuel Taylor Coleridge 1772-1834

Nurse Janet's Ethical Dilemma

Janet smiled to herself as she skipped across the concourse at Euston Station to catch the train north. She felt relaxed and happy; proud of her recent achievement. She had just completed her nurse training at St Thomas' Hospital; she had the nursing medallion in her pocket to prove it.

The final examination had been tough. There had been written papers, oral examinations, as well as the requirement to demonstrate her practical skills at the bedside. It had been an extremely stressful experience, but to her great relief she had passed, indeed she had passed with honours. She was now on her way home to celebrate with her family. No doubt her mother would make a fuss of her and invite all her friends round to share her good fortune. Then next week, she would return to London with her parents for the degree ceremony. After months spent studying for her exams, it would be a joyous occasion. She was looking forward to the pomp and ceremony, the mortarboard and ermine-lined gown and the inevitable celebratory party.

Her first post, as a newly qualified nurse, was to be on the children's ward at Lancaster's Royal Infirmary. She was a farmer's daughter, her home the nearby town of Kendal, and in her new job, she would be able to spend more time with her parents and rekindle old friendships recently neglected.

She was pleased to find a quiet carriage on the train and took a seat opposite a distinguished-looking gentleman and his rather dowdy, dumpy wife. Not being a regular churchgoer, she wasn't certain of his exact status but wearing a purple shirt and a clerical collar, he was clearly a 'man of the cloth'. A large silver cross on a heavy silver chain hung from his neck onto his portly chest. *Not a regular parish priest*, she thought, *probably a bishop*.

She said a polite 'Good Morning' and received a similar greeting in reply. Then, taking off her coat and placing it on the empty seat at her side, she retrieved a book from her bag, relaxed and began to read.

She felt at peace with the world as she settled back and watched the pleasant English countryside slide past, every mile, every minute, taking her closer to home. She had never been completely at ease in London with its hustle, bustle and noisy, crowded streets where everyone looked anxious and worn, too busy rushing around even to say a civil 'Good morning.' She was a country girl at heart, born to the slower pace of rural life, where there was always time to pass the time of day with a friendly neighbour, to remark on the weather, or simply to stop and admire the distant Lakeland hills, whose clothes changed seamlessly with the passing of the seasons; fresh and green in the spring, tinged with purple heather in autumn, white, forbidding and cold in winter.

Occasionally she glanced across at her travelling companions. The bishop was engrossed in the Times crossword but there was something vaguely familiar about his wife. Janet was certain she'd seen her somewhere before. But where? Had she perhaps been a patient she'd nursed in the hospital? If so, she couldn't recall her name or her medical complaint.

She returned to her book, but glanced up occasionally to take a furtive look at the woman sitting opposite, fortunately without attracting the attention of the bishop. Each time she took a surreptitious peek, the more certain she became that she knew her.

And then quite suddenly, it struck her. She hadn't seen this particular woman before, but she had seen a photo of a woman with a very similar face in one of her nursing textbooks. She could picture the page now; it was in the chapter on thyroid problems. If the thyroid gland was overactive, the patient was slim, anxious, and excitable with wide, staring eyes. The image in the nursing manual was of a woman with the opposite condition; that in which the thyroid was underactive; a disease called myxoedema.

In her mind, she recalled the features of the condition. Damn it, she should have recognised it sooner. There had even been a question on thyroid problems in her recent exam! It occurred predominantly in middle-aged women who tended to put on weight. She looked again at the bishop's wife and decided she fitted that description. What else did she know of the condition? Having revised recently for her final exam, she recalled all the signs and symptoms vividly. Thyroid patients tended to lose their hair, and their skin became dry and flaky. Again she glanced across the carriage and, now feeling excited, saw that this woman also had these features.

Janet also knew that these patients often had a large goitre or possibly a scar on the neck from a previous thyroid operation. But she couldn't see her neck; the bishop's wife was wearing a scarf. But of course, patients with this condition always felt the cold, and it certainly wasn't cold in the carriage. She wondered if somehow she could get the Bishop's wife to speak. Thyroid patients had a deep husky voice.

She decided to play detective. She opened the packet of sweets she was carrying, had one herself, then offered them to the lady hoping to hear her voice as she acknowledged the gift and offered her thanks. Irritatingly though, the bishop replied on his wife's behalf.

'That's very kind of you,' he said, in a deep and melodic voice that Janet could imagine resonating around a grand church or cathedral, 'but my wife doesn't eat sweets.' He patted his own generously proportioned abdomen as if to suggest that his wife was fat enough already.

Despite this setback, Janet remained certain of her diagnosis. She wondered if she ought to mention it to the bishop but, not wishing to cause any offence, her courage failed her.

The train rattled on through the Midlands, stopping at Rugby and then at Stoke on Trent, and still, Janet felt unable to raise the subject that was now worrying her. Surely the bishop would want to know if his wife was ill. But she told herself that it was none of her business, and once more tried to settle into her book.

But her conscience niggled, and unable to concentrate on her novel, she now remembered that patients with an underactive thyroid gland were at risk of coronary artery disease and heart attacks. Surely, with this knowledge, it wasn't simply right to speak to the Bishop, she had a moral responsibility to express her concern.

The train stopped at Crewe, then raced on across the Cheshire plain with its rich green pastures and scattered red brick farmhouses. Janet was torn with indecision. She had grave concern for the woman's health and began to fear that within a couple of weeks, she might perish from a massive heart attack. She knew she ought to speak to the bishop, yet still, her confidence still eluded her.

The final stop, at Stockport's Edgeley station, came and went and Janet knew they would arrive at Manchester's Piccadilly station in precisely five minutes time. It was now or never. It was her duty to speak out; it would be unethical, indeed totally irresponsible not to do so.

'Excuse me,' she said to the bishop, in a voice that was hesitant and barely audible.

'Yes, my dear, can I help you?' the bishop replied in his sonorous voice.

'Look, I know I'm speaking out of turn, and perhaps I shouldn't mention it, but I'm a nurse. I've just qualified, and I'm worried about your wife. I'm sure she has an underactive thyroid gland.

The bishop smiled gently. 'Yes, my dear. You're quite right,' he replied, glancing fondly at his wife. 'Before her operation, her thyroid gland was overactive, and she chattered incessantly. She was full of nervous energy. She chased me out of my office three times every day to polish, clean, and tidy it. It was like living in the middle of a hurricane with a hundred whirling dervishes and I couldn't get a moment's peace. My life was quite intolerable. The surgeon did a great job; things are so much easier now. The truth is that I prefer her this way.'

A Touch of Blarney

Working anxiously in Casualty at the City General Hospital during my first week as a doctor, I was completely unaware of the time, but it was already one in the morning.

I was tired and hungry. Seven long hours had passed since I'd had anything solid to eat; I'd survived on frequent mugs of sweet tea and the occasional biscuit.

I felt abused! Was this a foretaste of what my life would be like for the next twelve months? Fortunately, though, Bill, the night porter, and Stan, the night security guard, an ex-policeman, had dropped by and were cheerfully producing thick slices of hot buttered toast.

'That's a lovely smell,' my next patient said, in a soft Irish accent.

His nose was held up in appreciation of the aroma, reminding me of the boys in that well-known 'Aaah Bisto' gravy advertisement. His appearance suggested he was a tramp. He was dirty and unkempt, wore a faded, old gabardine raincoat and was holding a woollen hat, which I presumed to be responsible for the tidemark across his forehead. Below the line, his face was weather-beaten and brown; above the line, it was strikingly pale. He obviously spent much of his life outdoors, wearing his hat most of the time. He was carrying a mug of tea in his hand, which struck me as being unwise. Patients were advised not to eat or drink before they saw the doctor, lest an anaesthetic subsequently be required. Notices to this effect were prominently displayed throughout the department.

My initial 'foot of the bed' impression was that he didn't look particularly ill; in fact, he looked both healthy and cheerful. He appeared to be pleased with himself, for there was a hint of humour on his quizzical face and a sparkle in his eyes. I was surprised he'd been able to smell the buttered toast because the whiff that reached my nostrils was that of methylated spirits.

'Top of the morning to you, Doctor,' he said. 'To be sure 'tis a nice, clear, cold night, is it not?'

'You're Irish by the sound of it. Where exactly are you from?'

'I am indeed from Ireland,' he said. 'The Emerald Isle; God's own country, from a little village called Killybegs. It's right up in the north, in County Donegal. And a lovely spot it is too. Have you ever been there, Doctor?'

'Actually, I have,' I replied, recalling a holiday I'd enjoyed there with my parents, many years previously, 'and wild and beautiful it is. So what brought you to this country?'

'Tis a long story to be sure, but I'm a priest.'

I must have looked surprised as I tried to reconcile his present appearance with his stated calling. Then he continued, now in a confessional whisper.

'Well, Doctor, to tell you the truth, I used to be a priest, but I was a bit of a naughty boy. You see, I became a little over-fond of the communion wine, helping myself rather too freely. The Bishop of Donegal disapproved and sent me packing, not that he didn't partake of a tipple or two himself, you understand!'

An interesting character, I thought, *a defrocked priest, down on his luck.* I was tempted to delve deeper into his background but, conscious of the time and hoping to get a little sleep at some stage before morning, I decided to move the consultation along.

I asked him what the problem was.

'Tis my belly, Doctor, so it is.' he said, 'I've a terrible pain in my belly; it's as if there's a plague of rats in there, gnawing at my innards.'

He went on to describe his troubles in great detail, but it was a story that I found difficult to untangle. The site of the pain suggested it might be arising from the stomach, but he insisted it troubled him when he moved his arms into certain positions, and occasionally when he scratched his head. This was not a combination of symptoms with which I was familiar from my study of medical textbooks! He also described a pain behind his left eye, 'only my left eye mind, Doctor,' when he passed water, again an amalgam of symptoms I had not encountered in five years at medical school!

It took nearly ten minutes for him to undress to allow me to examine his abdomen because of the multiple layers of clothes he wore. When he had taken off his jacket, three ragged sweaters, and an old waistcoat, I thought we would soon be rewarded by the sight of flesh. However, the removal of a 'once white' grey vest and the remains of a shirt were required, (there were more holes in it than material holding it together) before we finally reached his skin.

Having achieved this objective, however, I discovered whilst examining his abdomen that his clinical signs were as perplexing as his symptoms! One minute the tenderness was on his left side, causing him to cry out and leap from the examination couch in an alarming fashion. The next minute, the pain seemed worse on the right. Yet, at other times, he would allow deep palpation without any apparent discomfort whilst happily relating stories of his beloved homeland. Half an hour later, the only conclusion I'd reached was that I didn't have a clue what was wrong with him!

It was at this moment that Sister Holman, who had run the department firmly but fairly for over twenty years and had the wisdom that results from experience, walked through the door. She beamed at my patient, 'Oh, it's you, Charlie. So you've decided to pay us another visit?'

'Sure I have, Sister, and can I say what a joy it is, to see your lovely happy smiling face once again.'

'Have you had yourself a cup of tea, Charlie?'

'Yes, thank you, Sister, a nice big mug. Hot and sweet and lovely it was too, brewed by one of your little angels.'

'Would you like another drink before you go?'

'By any chance, would there be some nice buttered toast with that, Sister?'

Sister smiled. 'Yes, Charlie, there would, provided that you promise not to come back.'

Then, rather more severely, she added, 'This is a hospital, Charlie, a place for the sick and infirm. It's not a port of call for ex-naval sea captains down on their luck.'

Finally, belatedly, it dawned on me that Charlie had succeeded in getting two free mugs of tea, some hot buttered toast, and had spent a couple of hours in a nice warm environment, whilst successfully pulling the wool over my naive eyes. However, his plan to spend the night between freshly laundered hospital sheets, and have a cooked breakfast in the morning had been thwarted.

'He's actually not an ex-navy captain tonight, Sister,' I said, 'he's a defrocked priest.'

'Is that so,' she said smiling, then turning to the patient, whom she obviously knew well, she added, 'in that case, Charlie, please say a prayer and a couple of Hail Marys for us whilst you are having that mug of tea, and then be on your way.'

'I will, Sister. I will. And I'll say one for the young doctor too. May the Good Lord bless you and keep you both safe and warm in His arms,' he said, ...'til I pop in and see you both again,' he added with a wink.

<u>Thought for the day</u>

What you take for lying in an Irishman is only his attempt to put a herbaceous border on stark reality.

Oliver St John Gregory 1878-1957

French Piles

'Frank, my piles are killing me. I need something to give me some relief. It was so stupid of me not to bring my ointment. I can't think how I forgot. Would you drive into that town we came through on the way here and see if you can pick something up at a chemist?'

'I'm not sure my French is up to that, but I'll give it a try.'

'The chemist is almost certain to speak English, most of them do over here, don't they? But, just in case, take that French phrase book with you and perhaps a paper and pencil as well.'

'You're surely not suggesting I draw a picture of your piles?'

'Well, yes I am, but only if there's no other way you can get him to understand. But it would probably better to ask if he has an English to French dictionary.

***

Frank: 'Bonjour.'

Pharmacist: 'Bonjour, Monsieur, comment puis-je vous aider?'

Frank: 'Ma femme, elle a les piles.'

Pharmacist: 'Je ne comprehend pas 'piles'. Quels sont les 'piles'?'

Frank (louder): 'Piles; tres grand piles.'

Pharmacist : 'Piles; qu'entendez-vous par 'piles'.
Le mot 'Piles' signifie 'Lots of'. Eh bien, votre femme a beaucoup de quoi? Beaucoup d'argent? Beaucoup d'enfants?'

Frank: 'Beaucoup de piles sur la derriere.'

Pharmacist: 'Beaucoup de derriere. Votre femme a un grand fond, un grand derriere?'

Frank: 'Non, non, non. Pas un large derriere. Well, actually, oui, she has un grande derriere mais le problem est un grand pile sur la grande derriere. Avez vous a dictionary?'

Pharmacist: 'Oui une dictionnaire. C'est une bonne idée. J'en ai une ici'

Frank: 'Regardez ici. Piles, elle a les piles.'

Pharmacist: 'Maintenant, je comprends. Hémorroïdes vous voulez dire. Hémorroïdes! Votre femme a des hémorroïdes.'

Frank:'Oui Haemorrhoids, tres large haemorrhoids sur la derriere. Beaucoup de mal.'

Phamacist: 'Saignent-ils?'

Frank: 'Non comprendo'

Pharmacis: 'They bleed, oui?'

Frank: 'Non bleed. Ils ne bleed pas. Mais ils sont tres grande et beaucoup de mal.'

Phamacist: 'J'ai des suppositoires qui aideront.'

Frank: 'Non. Pas suppositories. Ointment. Avez-vous some ointment?'

Pharmacist: 'Ointment, tu veux dire pommade. Oui, j'ai de la pommade. Je vais en obtenir pour vous. Appliquer quatre fois par jour.'

Frank: 'Oui, quatre times a day. Merci.'

Pharmacist; 'Dois-je envelopper pour vous?'

Frank: 'Je m'excuse. Non comprendo.'

Pharmacist: 'Voulez-vous me le mettre dans un sac?'

Frank: 'Oh, you mean, mettre in a bag. Non, il n'est pas necessary.'

Pharmacist: 'Eh bien ce sera douze euros s'il vous plaît.'

Frank: 'Ca, c'est cher n'est pas?'

Pharmacist: 'Oui, peut-être. Mais c'est un très bon onguent pour les piles.'

Frank: 'Merci beaucoup. Ma femme will be tres heureux. Je suis happy that we got there in the end.'

Pharmacist: 'I'm only too pleased to help. I hope you enjoy the rest of your holiday, and that your wife's piles clear up quickly. Don't hesitate to return if you need any further assistance.'

Thoughts for the day

No matter how politely or distinctly you ask a Parisian a question, he will persist in answering you in French.

Fran Lebowitz 1946

You know the trouble with the French, they don't even have a word for entrepreneur.

Attributed to George W. Bush 1946

Bridie

Mrs Bridget Conlon's job title at the hospital was Domestic Supervisor; her area of responsibility, the doctor's residency. She had held the job for as long as anyone could remember. Her job description stated that she was employed to manage all aspects of the catering and accommodation for the twenty or so young doctors for whom the residency was home. This comprised a dining room, a large lounge, two communal washrooms and a single room for each of the doctors.

However, in her heart, she knew that her principal role was not to manage the building and the services within it, but to guide the newly-qualified doctors safely through the rigours of their twelve-month internship. A giant of a woman with an equally large heart, she was fiercely protective of the young men and women in her care. She undertook the role of a mother hen, not by smothering them with kindness as a nurse might do with sick children, rather she applied the firm but fair hand of the regimental sergeant major.

Mrs Conlon ensured not only that the doctors were well-fed, but also that they took care of their own health. If they were summoned to deal with a sick patient whilst eating their evening meal, she would issue a stern rebuke.

'You'll be no use to your patients, young Lady,' she would say, 'if you rush your meal and give yourself an ulcer. Who's going to look after them if you become ill?'

And like a good mother, she was also capable of a stern reprimand; 'You let yourself down, young Sir, using language like that. You wouldn't be using words like that at home now, would you?'

Equally, any young doctor whose room was left untidy would be admonished and given an ultimatum; 'I want to see this room spick and span by dinner time... or else!'

Known to the young doctors as 'Bridie' she was loved and respected by them all.

Bridie was assisted by two young cleaners, Mary Murphy and Marie Maguire who hailed from County Mayo on the west coast of Ireland which, perhaps not by chance, happened to be Bridie's country of birth.

One day Mary and Marie, both good Catholic girls, came to speak with Bridie in a state of considerable distress.

'Mrs Conlon' they wailed, 'two of the doctors have gone and done a terrible thing. They've moved their two beds into one of their rooms and put the chairs and cupboards into the other.'

'And the names of the two doctors?'

'Dr Webster and Dr Potter in rooms 11 and 12. Side by side, the beds are, in room 12, Mrs Conlon. We're fearful worried for the doctors.'

'That would be Dr Anne Webster and Dr Bernard Potter. Well, please go immediately and replace the furniture as it ought to be. There will be no sinful hanky panky in the residency whilst I am in charge!'

When the two doctors returned to their rooms that evening, they were irritated to find that their convivial domestic arrangement had been disturbed.

'Where we place the furniture in our own rooms is our business and nobody else's,' Anne said.

'Agreed, those girls have a damn cheek,' Bernard replied, as they quickly reorganised things for their own convenience and pleasure.

The next day, the two doctors went about their duties on the wards as usual, only to find, to their great annoyance when the returned in the evening, that their two single beds had once more been placed in separate rooms.

On the third morning, Bridie, having again been alerted by Mary and Marie, went in person to investigate and was appalled to find the two beds snuggling side by side in room 12. Even more shocking, on further investigation, she found an empty silver foil packet in the wastepaper basket.

'Mother Mary, this is quite intolerable,' she muttered to herself as she again instructed her girls to return the furniture to its proper place. She was responsible for the building, for the standard of behaviour within it and this was conduct she simply would not allow.

The beds were moved to and fro, morning and evening, for two further days. All the while, Bridie, Mary, and Marie became more and more indignant that the two young doctors were living in sin, whilst the doctors became increasingly angry that the maids were creating work for them, undermining their cosy domestic arrangement, and telling them how to lead their lives.

Finally, Bridie decided the situation could not be tolerated any longer; enough was enough, action must be taken. It was, however, not a situation she had met before, and she was uncertain how best to proceed. Whilst determined to stop such wicked conduct, she lacked the confidence to confront the doctors face to face on a matter of such delicacy.

After due consideration, she decided it would be easier to write to them rather than risk an embarrassing verbal exchange. She then spent an agonising day drafting and redrafting a letter, reproaching them on their unholy behaviour, and reminding them of the Sixth of God's ten commandments 'Thou shalt not commit adultery'. When finally satisfied that the letter conveyed her displeasure and censure in suitable terms, she went to room 12, the one that had become a double bedroom. She planned to place her letter in a prominent position on the bedside cabinet where it could not possibly be overlooked.

However, when she opened the door, she was surprised to discover there was no space on the cabinet. The doctors had forestalled her by leaving a copy of their marriage certificate, two large framed photographs of their wedding day - and a couple of packets of Durex for good measure.

Thought for the day

Things have come to a pretty pass when religion is allowed to invade the sphere of private life.
Lord Melbourne 1779 - 1848

Doctor Regrets Stealing from His Patient

Dr Andrew Jackson knew the staff at the High Grove Medical Practice regarded him as being old fashioned, but he didn't care; in fact, the knowledge rather pleased him. He wasn't afraid to stand out from the crowd. The truth was that he hadn't taken kindly to the changes his younger colleagues had introduced in recent years. Of course, as the senior partner he could have prevented them had he chosen to do so, but accepting they would be running the surgery when he retired, he had allowed them free rein.

He liked to reminisce about the days when life was lived at a slower pace when there was more time to spend with patients. He hated the computer that now sat on his desk; how could he possibly give his whole attention to his patients, when he had to have one eye on the screen? And was he really expected to learn to type at his age? He resented the bureaucracy, the form-filling, the targets, and the endless 'top-down' imperatives that now ruled his life. And he cursed all those courses he was obliged to attend; courses on audit, equality, governance, algorithms, health and safety, fire regulations, and those wretched seminars on good communication. What a waste of time. Where had common sense gone? What could they tell him about communication that he hadn't practised every day for the last thirty-five years?

And why did everyone now call him 'Andy'? With hindsight, he realised that he ought to have insisted that his partners called him 'Andrew' and that the staff address him as 'Dr Jackson'. He sighed. It was too late now, of course; he would just have to accept it until he retired. Fortunately, he didn't have too long to wait, just a few more months.

In the meantime, he would do the things that he enjoyed best, which was spending time with his patients. Fortunately, caring for the old folk, or 'chronics', as they were often, but rather unkindly, referred to, was a job that others avoided; so he had been pleased to take on the task. That was why he now found himself in the warden-controlled flat belonging to Mary Taggart, an elderly lady whom he had known for many years. He'd cared for her husband when he had been dying with lung cancer, and over the years he'd delivered her daughter and two of her grandchildren. Now she was less of a patient, more of an old friend, and he was there to comfort her as she struggled with arthritis, diabetes, and early dementia.

'Hello again Mary,' he said, as he let himself in. 'And how are we today?'

Mary was sitting as usual in her easy chair, a small table at her side, on which were the items that formed the basis of her daily life; the morning newspaper, a library book, the remains of a cup of tea, a packet of sweets, a bowl of peanuts, and an ashtray containing the butts of numerous cigarettes. Guiltily, she covered the ashtray with the paper when Dr Jackson entered, but not before she had been spotted. In fact, the smell of stale cigarettes had permeated the carpets and was hanging heavily from the curtains and cushions, so her efforts were entirely in vain.

Mary brightened the moment she saw her visitor.

'Much the same as always, Doctor, but thank you for asking,' she said.

Dr Jackson knew that no medical decisions would be taken in the next fifteen minutes and that his partners would consider he was wasting his time, but he didn't care; for Mary, his visit would make this a special day.

'Still being a naughty girl, I see.'

Dr Jackson smiled as he spoke, he knew full well that to chide Mary or to give her a lecture on the dangers of smoking would be a waste of time; it would have no effect whatsoever!

'I'm so glad you've come, Doctor, I've something special to show you.'

With difficulty, she rose from her chair and, using her walking frame, pottered to the sideboard. She began rummaging in one of the drawers.

As Dr Jackson patiently waited for her to return, he spotted the peanuts. He glanced to see that Mary's back was turned and helped himself to a couple. They were the plain, non-salted ones that he preferred. Better for me, he thought, too much salt is bad for my hypertension.

'Dear, dear, now where can that photo be,' Mary muttered to herself. 'Perhaps it's next door.'

Slowly, Mary limped into the bedroom, and while she was out of the room, the doctor helped himself to a few more nuts; then a few more when he heard Mary shuffling about in the adjacent room.

'Look,' Mary said, when she finally returned, a contented smile on her face, 'a picture of Lisa, my granddaughter in her robes on her degree day. She qualified as a doctor last week. She's such a clever girl; I'm so proud of her. Do you remember the day you delivered her? You had to fight your way through a snowstorm to get there. Look, she's so grown up now.'

She handed the photo to the doctor.

'Now somewhere I've got a photo of her as a baby. I'm sure you'll want to see that too, Doctor, to see how much she's grown.'

She toddled off again, giving Dr Jackson time to help himself to a few more nuts. Then, to his horror, he realised that the bowl was now nearly empty. The chances were that, despite being somewhat forgetful and having poor eyesight, Mary would notice.

Mary returned with another photo, this time of her granddaughter as a bonny, one-year-old baby.

'Look how she's changed, Doctor. I can't believe that she's done so well.'

Dr Jackson admired the two photos, agreeing that Lisa had changed enormously. He could understand Mary's pride and asked that his congratulations be passed on to Lisa before adding, 'Look, Mary, I'm afraid that I've a confession to make. I've eaten a few of your peanuts. I'll bring another packet for you next time I come.'

'Oh, Doctor, there's no need for you to bother. My daughter brings me a new packet each week. She knows how much I like them. But since I lost my teeth, I just suck the chocolate off then throw the nuts away.'

Thought for the day

Opportunity makes a thief
13th century proverb

In Trouble with the Police

I had just taken delivery of a Triumph TR 2 Sports car. It wasn't new, of course, but it had still cost me the best part of a year's salary. Low, sleek, and streamlined, in British racing green, with wire wheels and leather upholstery, it was my pride and joy. Whenever off duty, I spent my time waxing the bodywork, polishing the chrome and tinkering under the bonnet. Nothing was more enjoyable on a warm summer's evening than to speed along some quiet country road, the hood down, the wind in my face, enjoying the admiring glances of envious folk as I raced passed.

Bill Smith, a pal of mine who worked at the eye hospital, was just one of the many friends and colleagues who asked to be taken for a spin in the car, and of course, it was my pleasure to oblige them. On this particular Saturday, we were bowling along in the early evening sunshine on the A5 between Lake Bala and Bangor in North Wales. This mountain road with its hill climbs and tight bends could have been designed for the TR 2. It offered every opportunity to demonstrate the car's agility, acceleration, and road-holding ability. Feeling elated, smiles on our faces, we gobbled up the miles, the twin-carburettor, four-cylinder engine, tuned to 90 bhp, purring along beautifully; and the coil-springed suspension giving us the smoothest of rides.

'How fast will she go?' Bill asked.

'The top speed recorded for the TR2 is over 120 mph,' I said, 'but that's for the souped-up version; the one they use in the RAC rallies. The TR2 has won that event more than once you know. This is the roadster model - top speed, 107 mph.'

'Well, go on then,' he replied.

I needed no further encouragement! On the next straight stretch, I pressed the accelerator pedal hard to the floor. I felt the G force, the seat pressing into my back, as the car rocketed forward. The speedometer registered 70, then 80 mph. With the roar of the engine, the squeal from the tyres as we took a slight bend and the countryside whizzing past, it was exhilarating stuff. As we reached 90 mph, I was suddenly aware of a motorcycle on our tail. My heart sank it was a police bike! Gently I applied the Lockheed drum brakes and slowed the car. The police bike overtook us and then indicated that we should stop.

I pulled into the next lay-by, and the policeman parked some 20 yards in front. Slowly he got off his bike, kicked down the stand, and turned to face us. For a moment, he just stood there looking at us, his hands on his hips. Slowly, almost casually, he raised his goggles, leaving them resting on his forehead. Then very deliberately, finger by finger, he removed one gauntlet, followed by the second, before positioning them carefully on the seat of his bike. In a leisurely fashion, he took off his helmet and tucked it under his arm. We were guilty. We knew it, he knew it, and he was going to take pleasure in putting us in the book! There was a malevolent gleam in his eye and the suggestion of a smile on his face, as he walked slowly towards us.

'We're in trouble now,' I said.

'Maybe not,' Bill whispered. 'Just let me do the talking.'

He stopped a couple of yards short of the bonnet, pausing before reaching into his jacket pocket and producing a small notebook. He caught my eye and smiled malignly, enjoying my discomfort, before slipping his hand into a second pocket and pulling out a pencil. He licked its tip and then carefully recorded our registration number in his notebook.

Reaching the driver's door, the policeman cast his eye along the length of the car, noting its smooth lines and beautifully polished paintwork. *If his own car is a rusty, old banger*, I thought, *he'll be particularly vindictive.*

Then he spoke, his voice cold and sarcastic. 'Don't tell me - let me guess. Your house is on fire, and you're racing home to save it.'

'No, Officer,' I muttered.

'Well, perhaps you've just heard that your wife is in labour and you're rushing to the maternity unit.'

'No, Officer.'

'In that case, do please tell me why you were driving at 90 mph. You do know what the speed limit is, I suppose?'

'Yes, Officer, 60mph.'

'You were doing 90; that's 30 mph over the limit.' His voice hardened. 'I'm going to throw the book at you. You won't be driving this fancy car of yours for many years to come. By the time I've finished with you, your driving license will be suspended, you'll get a hefty fine, and with any luck, you'll receive a good long prison sentence as well.'

Then Bill spoke for the first time, his voice calm, the words clear and unhurried. 'Do let me explain, Officer. I realise we were over the speed limit, and I apologise for that, but please don't blame my driver. You see, I work at the eye hospital in Wrexham; look, I have my identification badge here.'

He dived into his pocket and presented the policeman with his hospital badge inscribed with his photo, his name, and department.

'I work as part of the corneal transplant service. There was a death at the Wrexham's Maelor Hospital this morning, and I'm delivering an eye that is required in Bangor. I'm sure you'll understand that if the transplant is to be successful, speed is of the essence. Look, I have it here.'

He unzipped his bag and produced a sealed glass tube the size of a small jam jar. It containing clear liquid and floating in the fluid was an eye.

As Bill lifted it up to show the policeman, the eye floated around the jar in a disconcerting manner.

'As I said, Officer, time is of greatest importance, so I would be obliged if we could get on our way.'

The policeman's reaction was at first shock, then dismay as he realised he wouldn't have the pleasure of booking us for speeding. The last thing he wanted on his conscience was responsibility for a failed transplant. He looked again at the eye, which stared back at him in a baleful fashion.

'OK, right,' he stuttered. 'Perhaps you would like me to escort you to Bangor to save you any further hold-ups.'

'That's very thoughtful of you, Officer,' Bill replied, as cool as you like, 'but that won't be necessary, the roads are quiet at the moment, but as I say, we really mustn't delay any longer.'

Reluctantly, the policeman returned to his bike, and I started the engine and pulled back onto the road. As we continued on our way, I asked Bill if it really was a human eye.

'No, of course not! It's a sheep's eye. I got it from the butcher. It's pickled in formalin. This is the second time it's helped me to avoid a speeding ticket.'

'That policeman looked ever so disappointed that he couldn't book us,' I commented.

'Yes,' Bill replied. 'But it serves him right for being so officious and telling lies. He was right out of order; there's no way you can be sent to prison for speeding.'

'No,' I replied, 'but they can for perverting the course of justice!'

An Unlikely Story

'Your next patient seems to have come with her own bodyguard. You'd better not take any liberties with her!'

It was Sally, the diminutive staff nurse, who offered Toby the advice. The accident department was busy, as was usually the case late on a Saturday evening. Toby, deputising for the regular casualty officer who was on annual leave, was working his way through a backlog of cases. It had been a long day, and he was tired and irritable.

'What seems to be her problem?' he asked, looking up from the notes he was writing on a lad who had sprained his ankle playing football earlier in the day.

'I'm not sure. She doesn't look very ill, and her observations are fine, but she's clutching her belly in a very theatrical fashion. The fellow with her is an ugly brute of a man, and he's getting aggressive because she's been kept waiting. She's in the middle cubicle.'

'It would be nice to see a proper case, someone with some genuine pathology. I'm fed up of treating patients with minor scratches, trivial bruises, and vague belly ache who ought to be to be sorted out by their GPs. That's all I've seen all day,' Toby grumbled.

'Count yourself lucky,' Sally responded. 'Last night, we had a woman call in because she'd run out of her contraceptive pills. Beat that for cheek!

Fancy coming into an accident and emergency department simply because she wanted a bit of nooky!'

'I hope you sent her away with a flea in her ear.'

'I didn't, but Sister certainly did! She went away, very frustrated! I bet her fellow was too, when she got home and told him the news.'

Wearily, Toby set aside his mug of tea, picked up his stethoscope, and went to see the patient.

As he pulled aside the cotton screen that served as a door to the cubicle, the young woman sitting on the examination couch clutched her abdomen and groaned dramatically. She was wearing a miniskirt that was little more than a pelmet, and a diaphanous white blouse, through which a black bra was clearly visible. A smell of cheap perfume and alcohol filled the cubicle, disguising the odour of

116

hospital antiseptic, which normally pervaded the air.

Toby glanced at her casualty card and then introduced himself. The woman's name was Susan Haines; she wore no ring.

'Hello, Miss Haines. What seems to be the problem?'

'It's the same problem I was here with a couple of days ago, Doctor, only now it's ten times worse.'

She obviously expected Toby to have her previous attendance record.

'I'm afraid I don't have the notes of that visit,' he explained, 'so just tell me the story from the start.'

Her companion interrupted aggressively.

'Well, you damn well ought to have them. What sort of a bloody hospital is this?'

'Did you tell the receptionist you were here a few days ago?' Toby asked innocently, knowing that had they done so, the notes would have been made available to him.

'They didn't bother to ask!' came the gruff reply.

Toby turned back to his patient, 'OK,' he said, 'the story from the beginning please.'

'I were at the flicks with me boyfriend, watching a film; that one 'bout a fire in a skyscraper. We was sharing some crisps an' I felt sommut solid in me mouth. He were messing 'bout with me at the time,' she said, indicating the man at her side, 'and I went an' swallowed it, didn't I? Whatever it were, must 'ave come from the packet of crisps. The minute I swallowed it, I were in pain. Horrid it were. It were like a red hot poker in the middle of me chest, just here, behind me breast bone. Since then, the pain has travelled ever so slow like. It's now behind me belly button. When I were 'ere last, the doctor x-rayed me and said 'e thought it were a jagged piece of glass. It's obviously movin' through me system and cutting into me guts. I really am in agony, Doctor. I'm terrified of the damage it's doing to me. Truly, I fear for me life.'

Her boyfriend was stocky and muscular. His head was clean-shaven and there was a tattoo on the side of his neck. Wearing braces over a grubby T-shirt, he looked like a bouncer from one of the local night clubs; not the sort that Toby would care to meet, late at night, in one of the dark alleys that surrounded the hospital. He reinforced her story.

'She's bin in agony, Doc. You'd best sort it out,' he said. The words, roughly spoken, accompanied by a finger jabbing pointedly at Toby's face, sounded threatening.

Toby examined Susan's abdomen carefully. As he did so, she 'oohh'd and aahh'd' impressively and periodically jumped violently as if a tender spot had been pressed; but the site of these painful areas was not consistent. When he subsequently returned to press the same spot a second time, there was little reaction at all. Toby judged that her tenderness was grossly exaggerated. It seemed unlikely the piece of glass had done any internal damage.

He took her pulse, blood pressure, and temperature. As Sally had said, these were all normal, adding to Toby's view that Miss Haines was not particularly ill, despite her dramatics and obvious concern. Nonetheless, since the glass was sufficiently dense to be visible on x-ray, he decided it would be a sensible precaution to x-ray her again, to see if it had moved down the bowel.

'I think we'll have another x-ray,' he said. 'Very often things we swallow pass through the bowel from top to bottom if we give them enough time. An x-ray will show us how far down it's got.'

By the time she came back from the x-ray department an hour later, the receptionist had produced her previous attendance card. This confirmed the pain initially had been in the central part of her chest but, contrary to what she had told Toby, the x-ray report stated that no abnormality had been found. In particular, no foreign body had been seen.

Toby put the latest set of x-rays on the viewing box in the office. They appeared to be quite normal; he looked carefully for any sign of glass but could find none. He wondered whether it would be wise to admit Miss Haines for observation, but decided it would be safe to let her go home and ask her to attend again should there be any further problems. He returned to the patient, rather hoping the belligerent boyfriend might have become impatient and gone home; unfortunately though he was still hovering protectively at her side.

'I've had a look at your x-rays' he explained, 'and I'm pleased to say that they look normal.'

'That ain't right,' the boyfriend interjected; 'the last doctor said there were some glass inside 'er and she's still in pain; in fact, she's bin in agony. Them tablets that she were given last time 'aven't touched it.'

'Since you were here last,' Toby explained, 'the first set of films have been seen by the experts in the x-ray department, and they have decided they were clear. But you must understand that although bits of metal or objects made of thick glass do generally show up on x-rays, the fact that the x-rays are normal doesn't mean there's no glass present. Many pieces of wood, plastic, and some types of glass may not be dense enough to show up on an x-ray film.

What I suggest is that you go home, and come back if anything new develops.'

Toby turned to the patient. 'It would also be sensible to sieve your stools. I know that's not a pleasant task, but when the glass comes out, you'll be able to see what it was, and you'll have the satisfaction of knowing that it's safely passed out of your body.'

The patient accepted this advice readily enough and seemed pleased at the prospect of returning home, but her minder was less happy.

'You mean she's to go sifting through her shit. That's not hygienic, Doc. It ain't right. That glass will be shredding her innards. She could be dead by morning for all you care. She needs to be kept in the hospital where she'll be safe. Then the nurses can do the dirty work. I'm warning you; you're going to be big trouble if she comes to any 'arm. There'll be all hell to pay if she dies; you mark my words, Doc.'

He looked pointedly at Toby's name badge. 'Thompson' he read. 'I'll remember that name, Thompson. Yer white coat an' posh voice won't protect you if I 'ave to come after you! You'll need to get yerself a lawyer.... and a bloody bodyguard,' he added as an afterthought, jabbing a finger into Toby's chest.

To cover himself, Toby reiterated that she should return if any further problems developed. He was pleased when the couple departed.

The boyfriend's parting shot as they left the department caused Toby considerable concern. He hoped he had done the right thing in allowing her to go home. Perhaps it would have been wiser to keep her in hospital overnight. Playing it safe wouldn't have cost him anything, and he would have avoided the sleepless night he would now endure, worrying that the patient might collapse and die at home. His anxiety would have been even greater had he known that in due course, he would have further dealings with this couple.

*****

A week later, Toby was surprised to see a face he recognized. He never ceased to marvel at the power of the human brain which has locked inside it, thousands of different memories, the details of which are released the moment the appropriate key is applied. The key may be a word, a gesture, or perhaps even a smell, but in this case, it was the patient's face and miniskirt. Toby recalled every detail of their previous encounter. It was brassy young Susan Haines.

As before, she was accompanied by her boyfriend, the heavily-built, tattooed and surly young man, who had made a point of noting Toby's name and had threatened him with violence. Also in the cubicle were her casualty attendance cards, now four in number, neatly stapled together. The information on the cards spoke of repeated attendances, with the site of her searing pain gradually moving lower, as if affected by gravity. On this occasion, however, she was no longer doubled up in agony; instead, she had a huge beaming smile on her face.

'I've passed it, Doctor,' she said triumphantly, as she held up a large, thick and jagged piece of glass. Toby looked at it with interest, his suspicions about this couple growing ever stronger in his mind. It appeared to be the major part of the rim of a glass milk bottle. It was three-quarters of an inch long, triangular in shape with a razor-sharp edge. Toby found it impossible to accept it would be possible to swallow such a large irregular object, let alone believe that a jagged piece of glass could pass along the entire length of her gut, without causing a blockage or a perforation on the way.

'My God, that must have caused you a great deal of pain when you passed it into the toilet,' he remarked.

'It was agony, Doctor. It took half an hour to pass, and I bled like a stuffed pig afterward.'

This stretched Toby's imagination just a little too far.

'You better let me have a look,' he said, 'to make sure you've not done any damage to your backside. If you turn onto your side, I'll get a little telescope and check for you.'

Immediately, her boyfriend stepped into the conversation. 'She don't need no examination, Doc,' he said in a gruff voice. 'She's fine now, and she don't want you messin' 'er about. You jus' needed to see what's caused all 'er troubles. We're going to complain to the company that made them crisps. That piece of glass could really 'ave damaged 'er; might even 'ave been the death of 'er. There ain't no way that summat like should 'ave been mixed in with them crisps. As it is, she's 'ad weeks of pain, she's lost money 'cos she's been off work, and she's come to casualty dozens of times; not that anyone 'ere's done a bloody thing to help 'er!'

It was quite clear in which direction the matter was proceeding. The couple intended to sue the manufacturer of the crisps and attempt to obtain compensation.

Toby turned to the girl. 'Are you sure you don't want me to check for any damage?'

Again it was the boyfriend who answered, his voice loud and aggressive, 'I've bloody told you already; she's sore enough as it is without any bloody tom-fool doctor poking about.'

Toby thought quickly. It was impossible to conceive that anyone could swallow such a large and jagged piece of glass whether sitting in daylight at the kitchen table or indeed on the back seat of a darkened cinema, no matter how distracted she might have been by her boyfriend's advances. She would have felt it in her mouth and, even if she had managed to swallow it, an obstruction or perforation of the gullet must surely have followed. It was far too large to reach the stomach, let alone pass through the entire length of the bowel.

'Look,' he said, 'it sounds as if you are going to contact the company, and I've no doubt they will then write to us. They're going to need a medical report to learn of all the problems you've had: the pain, the discomfort, and the bleeding from the back passage. They'll also need to confirm that you've attended the hospital on numerous occasions. Would it be best if we kept the piece of glass as evidence on your behalf?'

There was no immediate reply, as the two of them exchanged a glance. They considered the suggestion for a while. Eventually, it was the girl who replied.

'Yes, I think that would be best,' she said, but as she spoke, she looked for confirmation from the boyfriend, who nodded in agreement.

'Excellent,' Toby said, taking the piece of glass from her. 'I'm pleased to see you've given it a good wash! We'll keep it as evidence, and I'll make sure it's kept safe with your notes. When we hear from the crisp manufacturers, we'll write a report for them; we may even send this piece of glass to them as proof. I'm pleased it's all ended satisfactorily, and that you've not come to any serious harm.'

And so the consultation ended. Toby heaved a sigh of relief; with any luck, he wouldn't be seeing either of them again. But after the couple had departed, he decided to do some detective work. He taped the piece of glass securely to an investigation card and sent it to the x-ray department, requesting that they assess its radiodensity. He also asked for a review of all the x-rays that had been taken during the patient's recent attendances at the hospital.

He was not surprised a few days later, to receive a report from Dr Digby, the consultant radiologist, confirming that the piece of glass was extremely dense and would undoubtedly have shown up on her x-rays. He also confirmed that there was no evidence of any such foreign body on any of the series of four x-rays that had been taken. He added a note stating it was unfortunate that the patient had subjected herself to unnecessary exposure to x-irradiation, which was known to increase the risk of cancer. Toby made sure that all this additional evidence was included in the casualty record, and awaited the request for medical information from the crisp manufacturers that he anticipated would arrive very soon.

***

It was a month later that Mr Willoughby Scott, the Consultant Surgeon, took Toby to one side.

'Now Thompson, there's something I've been meaning to speak with you about,' he said, opening an envelope that had been in his pocket. Toby's heart immediately skipped a beat, wondering what he had done wrong. Why he asked himself, was he always plagued by self-doubt. But he needn't have worried.

'I'm sure you will remember this.'

He held up the thick piece of glass that Toby had taped to a casualty card some weeks previously.

Toby looked at it with interest. 'I certainly do. Have the manufacturers asked you to write a medical report, Sir?'

'Yes, they have, and as a result, I've reviewed the notes and x-rays taken on her various attendances in casualty. You were absolutely right. Come with me, and I'll show you.'

He led Toby down the corridor to his office. There were several piles of notes, both on the desk and on the floor, but the consultant quickly found the set he wanted and placed the relevant x-rays on the large viewing box that was mounted on the wall.

'This is the x-ray taken of the piece of glass the patient says she swallowed, using the same exposure that would have been employed for an abdominal or chest x-ray. You can see how dense it is. There can be no doubt it would have shown up on the x-rays taken in casualty, had it really been inside her body. I don't believe for one minute it was in a packet of potato crisps, and I agree with you, it looks like the rim of a milk bottle. Unquestionably, this is an attempt at compensation fraud. You've probably saved the company quite a lot of money. It was quick-witted of you to hang on to the glass and do the detective work.'

'Perhaps I shall get a lifetime's supply of potato crisps as a reward,' Toby commented, tongue in cheek.

'Probably not,' Mr Scott replied, smiling 'but if they did, they wouldn't do you any good. They're nothing but fat and salt, you know.'

'Do you feel that the police should be informed, Sir?'

Mr Scott considered the question for a moment. 'Yes, probably – but I think that's something for the crisp manufacturers to pursue. They were the intended victims of the fraud. If they do, I've no doubt that we will be asked for a witness statement.'

Toby had never written such a report; it was something upon which he might need some guidance.

'And would that be something I would be required to provide, or would you do it as the consultant in charge?'

'I am not entirely sure,' responded Mr Scott, 'but we'll cross that bridge when we come to it."

As it happened, Toby wasn't asked to write a report, indeed, he never heard anything more about the case. As Mr Saeed, the Registrar, explained to him later, if a report was requested, Mr Scott would undoubtedly write it himself and charge a fee of at least 100 guineas!

Thought for the day

O what a tangled web we weave
When first we practice to deceive

Sir Walter Scott 1771 -1832

A Lifelong Ambition

Jimmy was 28 years old when I first met him. He was good looking, 5 feet 10 inches tall, slightly built and a keen football fan - but he was also a violent criminal with severe mental health problems. Arrested, tried, and found guilty of causing grievous bodily harm, he received a custodial sentence. Later, he was referred to our secure mental health unit for attempts to be made to treat his aggressive behaviour.

I was tasked with working with him, and during one of our sessions, I asked what he would most like to achieve in his life?

His reply surprised me. 'To run a marathon,' he said.

I thought quickly. Was that practical, given that it was our responsibility to hold Jimmy in a secure environment, and avoid risk to the public?

'Yes, that might be possible,' I replied guardedly, 'but approval from your consultant will be required, and I would have to accompany you while you train.'

Fortunately, a couple weeks later, authorisation was forthcoming. It was hoped that sport and exercise might enable Jimmy to channel his aggression in a positive way.

Jimmy was really excited; for the first time in his life, he had an ambition he genuinely wished to fulfil that was achievable.

I suggested that a step-by-step approach should be adopted, with a marathon as the final objective, and we agreed that a local 10-kilometre run would be an acceptable start. Jimmy agreed, and training started in earnest.

His enthusiasm to run a marathon was set as a specific goal in his medical management programme, and it formed a major part of his rehabilitation. Whatever training I asked him to do, I did as well, often running up the 'Hill of Happiness'. We called it the Hill of Happiness as we were always happy to get to the top! Up and down involved a three kilometre run and a climb of 450ft.

We trained together, come rain, wind or shine, and six months later, we entered a 10-kilometre race for '*Dreams*' his chosen charity. This is a charity which helps children with serious and life-limiting conditions to fulfil a dream. We crossed the finish line, side by side, in just over an hour. Jimmy's consultant allowed us to have a celebratory pint in the local pub afterward. He agreed that Jimmy had earned the right to sit in the sun, in the pub garden and feel the precious gift we all take for granted; to be in control of your own life and have people who believe in you at your side. That moment was great, but it was just a foretaste of what was to come.

With his newfound confidence, Jimmy once feared for his aggression, started to play football for Norton Nomads, our mental health team. He was already physically fit, and the training we had done together helped with our unique bond. He knew I would be displeased if he was guilty of any violent conduct on the pitch.

People thought he would be sent off in his first match, but in the two seasons he played, he didn't pick up a single yellow card for a bad tackle, foul, or for verbal abuse. On one occasion, we played a high profile cup game at the local stadium. Afterward, the referee reported to the Football Association, that our mental health team had put the opposition to shame. We subsequently received a letter from the F A congratulating us on our respectful and honest play.

Jimmy went on to obtain 'A' level success in English and Maths. He got married and completed a three-year degree course in social work and social care.

I was proud of his success, and of my contribution to it, but for me, the moment that stood out and will stay with me for the rest of my life, was Jimmy's farewell game for the Norton Nomads, again played at the local Stadium, before he went to university. He brought his wife and parents along to watch him play. It was a friendly match, played for charity against a team of local celebrities, their friends and supporters. We played on opposite sides, and as the final whistle approached, the score was three goals each. Then his team was awarded a corner. The ball came across, and Jimmy soared in the air and headed the winner. As he rushed to celebrate with his teammates, he looked over to the crowd and waved to his family, before running back to restart the game.

That was my moment. We had competed against each other as we jumped together; he attempting to score, me trying to stop him. He won that little tussle and his team won the match. Whilst my team mates showed their disappointment at losing, I felt the satisfaction of success. I watched him as he celebrated. I will never forget the look of joy on his face when he scored that goal and the way he acknowledged his family.

It had been a long, hard, and at times a painful struggle for him to win through to that moment. People had doubted him; they'd said he would fail and yet there he was; a changed person. This is what the NHS did for this individual and, for me; it was the moment that made everything worthwhile.

I often wonder who helped who, at the end of our time together. To be honest, we both helped each other and did things we both would not have dreamed possible. From an initial meeting trying to find common ground, we ended up running 10k, winning the local knock-out Cup Competition and finally playing and beating Manchester United's mental health team at Old Trafford in front of Wayne Rooney.

(Based on a story by Paul Willis. 'Jimmy' is a pseudonym).

Thought for the day

To cure the mind's wrong bias, spleen
Some recommend the bowling green,
Some hilly walks, all, exercise!
Matthew Green 1696 - 1737

A Yorkshire Obituary

Farmer George Braithwaite and his wife Gladys had been happily married for 50 years when, quite suddenly, Gladys died. George was heartbroken, but being a practical man, he went to the funeral directors to make the appropriate arrangements, then visited the offices of The Yorkshire Post regarding an obituary.

When informed of the cost, George spluttered and in true Yorkshire fashion asked, 'How much?!!'

'I want summat simple,' he explained, reluctantly producing his wallet. 'My Gladys was a good-hearted and hard-working Yorkshire lass, but she wunt 'ave wanted 'owt swanky.'

'Perhaps a small poem', suggested the woman behind the desk.

'Nay,' George replied, 'she wunt 'ave wanted anything la-di-da. Just put; Gladys Braithwaite died.'

'But you need to say the date on which she died,' the secretary said.

'Do I? Well, put died 17th Jan 2016. That'll do nicely.'

'It's usual for the bereaved to add some meaningful phrase about the dearly departed.'

George considered for a moment. 'Well put, 'Sadly missed'. That'll do,' he said.

'You can have another four words,' he was told.

'No, no,' George cried, 'she never would 'ave wanted me to splash out; she wasn't that sort of woman.'

'The words are included in the price,' he was informed.

'Oh, are they? You mean I've paid for 'em?'

'Yes, indeed.'

'Well, if I've paid for 'em, I'm 'avin 'em.'

The obituary was duly printed as follows:

Gladys Braithwaite died, 17th January 2016. Sadly missed. Also Tractor for Sale.

Thought for the day

As invariably happens after one has passed forty, the paper sagged open at the obituary page.

S. J. Perelman 1904 - 1979

Annie Arnell

Annie Arnell had a morbid fear of hospitals. This was the result of an unfortunate accident she had as a 6-year-old. Eager to help her mother with the cooking, she had reached up and inadvertently pulled a pan of boiling water off the stove. She suffered severe scalds to her left arm, shoulder, and to the side of her chest. Weeks of hospitalisation followed, as well as numerous painful dressings and a number of skin grafts. Now, as a 25-year-old married woman, the sight of white-tiled walls and the smell of antiseptic haunted her, and this was what prevented her from seeking medical advice when she became pregnant.

For the first four months of her pregnancy, Annie refused to go to the antenatal clinic, despite her husband's entreaties. She wouldn't even consult her own doctor. As a result, she suffered her troublesome early morning sickness in silence. It was only when her heartburn, nausea, and sickness became more severe that she finally relented.

Sue, the midwife, welcomed her new patient to the Antenatal Clinic, introduced herself and after initial pleasantries, got down to the business of assessing Annie's condition. Discovering that, by dates, Annie was already twenty weeks pregnant, Sue gently chided her for not coming sooner, but was sympathetic and forgiving when the reason for the delay was explained.

'Never mind,' she said. 'No harm done; better late than never.'

Fortunately, apart from the sickness, there was nothing in the history or examination to suggest anything was amiss, and in due course, an ultrasound scan was performed. This suggested that Annie's baby was a girl but that she was at least twenty-four weeks pregnant.

'Do you and your husband want to know the sex of your baby,' she was asked.

'Yes please; it will be so much easier if we know.' came the reply.

'It looks very much as if you're going to have a girl, but she seems more advanced than 20 weeks. Are you sure of your dates?'

'Yes, absolutely sure.'

'Well, we'll scan you again at your next visit. We should be certain of your baby's sex by then, and we'll also have a better idea when we can expect your baby to arrive.'

A month later, a second scan was performed which confirmed that the baby was a girl, but equally, there was now no doubt that the pregnancy was at least four weeks more advanced than Annie had thought.

When told, Annie turned pale and looked shocked.

'Oh my God,' she whispered, 'I've gone and married the wrong man!'

Thought for the day

If men had to have babies, they would only ever have one each.
Diana, Princess of Wales 1961- 1997

A Memorable Postage Stamp

'Please will you lend me a stamp, Dad?'

I grinned; my lad often says 'lend' when he means 'give'!

'Yes,' I replied, 'they're in the usual place; behind the clock in the sitting room.'

'Yes, I've looked there, but they're all second-class stamps. I need a first-class stamp.'

'First Class? That's unusual. What's it for?'

'It's for my application for medical school. It needs to arrive by tomorrow morning.'

Normally, I would have chided him for leaving it so late but I couldn't. I was delighted.

'Just wait here for a moment,' I said, 'I'll see if I can find one.'

***

Our family name is Haigh. Apparently, the name traces its history back to the Middle Ages when Britain was inhabited by the Anglo-Saxons. It's derived from the Old English word 'haga', which means 'dweller by the haw or hedge'. You won't find many Haighs in the South East, Wales, or in Scotland, but in Yorkshire they're two a penny, particularly in the West Riding. Presumably, hedges were used to define ownership of land and to enclose animals before the industrial revolution and the development of the woollen mills.

My father was one of five children brought up in Huddersfield, and the only one brave enough to cross the Pennines and settle in Lancashire. He worked in the Treasurer's office in the Town Hall, so I was fortunate to have a middle-class upbringing, living in a semi-detached house in a residential suburb. However, this was 1948, shortly after the end of the Second World War, when life was tougher than it is now. Austerity in those days was real. Meat, coal, and clothing were rationed. Breakfast was bread on which jam had been spread and then scraped off; you walked to school and looked forward to the bottle of milk you were given midmorning. In winter, you went to bed wearing your vest and woke to find frost on the inside of your bedroom window.

Even as the forties became the fifties, and life became easier, Dad remained a Yorkshire man at heart and kept his native Yorkshire values. He watched the pennies carefully and *'waste not – want not'* was his favourite expression. He could make a roast chicken last 4 meals; hot roast on a Sunday, cold meat salad on the Monday, then mince and mash on Tuesday, and finally, a soup made from boiling the bones on Wednesday. It was Thursday before we needed to open a tin of spam or corned beef! On one memorable occasion, he even ground the dried chicken bones with a mortar and pestle and made a disgusting grey paste, which he flavoured with tomato ketchup. We ate it with boiled potatoes and root vegetables. Whenever we had a joint of meat, he collected the fat so that we could have bread and dripping sandwiches, which, flavoured with salt and pepper, were extremely tasty, though probably very high in cholesterol.

Another of my father's expressions was, *'you don't get ought for nought',* but this was a maxim he didn't always follow. If the rag and bone man passed with his horse and cart, he dashed out with a bucket and spade to collect any droppings, much to my mother's embarrassment. He also had a friend who worked for the blood transfusion service, from whom he obtained pints of time-expired human blood, which, together with the horse dung, he spread on his vegetable patch. These were the days when blood was regarded as being clean, before the dangers of hepatitis and HIV were appreciated.

My father passed his thriftiness to me, but whether this was nature or nurture, I cannot say. As a child, I preferred to save my pocket money rather than spend it. Dad wouldn't allow me to be a weekday paperboy; he didn't want it to interfere with my schooling, but I delivered papers at the weekend and in the school holidays. I also earned extra money by cutting the neighbour's hedges and lawns, quite hard work in the days of hand shears and push lawnmowers. Dad encouraged me to open a Post Office Savings Account, and once a week, I would visit the local Post Office and invest my earnings.

Christmas was always profitable; there were presents, of course, and as I got older, money earned from delivering Christmas Post. On Christmas Day, there was always a family party at Grandad Haigh's house. After a wonderful Christmas dinner, roast turkey with all the trimmings, we had a great time playing games and singing carols around the tree. My Grandad Haigh was a good pianist and had a fine voice. Then in return for a whiskery kiss from my Granny, I would be given a £5 note, the ones that were half the size of a newspaper and covered in bold curly black writing. I would have liked to add the note to my Post Office Savings, but my father always relieved me of it, *'for safekeeping'*, he used to say.

Years passed in a whirlwind of activity, working and worrying; marriage and mortgages, then the trials and tribulations of raising a family. As a child, my thrift had no particular purpose, but when I had children of my own, I determined my frugality should benefit them. What I wanted above all else, was something that had not been possible for me: a university education. Surely it is the responsibility of all parents to give their offspring every opportunity to better themselves? How proud and pleased I would be if one of my children were to qualify as a doctor, lawyer, engineer, or architect.

Memories of my childhood days had long gone when I was clearing out the attic one wet weekend many years later. And there it was, in a cardboard box of old school exercise books, hidden under some dust sheets, the small, grey account book with the bold purple writing on the front; my 'Post Office Savings Account', the record of my schoolboy activity. Idly, I opened it and flicked through the pages. It covered a period of three or four years and recorded the details of my regular, small, weekly investments: a shilling here, sixpence there and, at the time of my birthday, five shillings or more. My mind flashed back to the days of my childhood: school friends, memories of our family home, my parents, now sadly departed, the shopping, gardening, and all the other little jobs I did to earn money. I turned to the last page. Most of the money, over six pounds, had been withdrawn on a day in June 1958. I wondered what I'd bought with it, perhaps a new bike, but couldn't remember. But I noticed that 13 shillings and sixpence remained in the account. What I asked myself, would 30 years compound interest be on 13 shillings and sixpence? Probably not very much, but I decided it would be fun to pop into a Post Office one day and find out.

'I've never seen one of these before', said the young girl behind the counter, when I presented the Savings Account Book to her and asked to withdraw my money, together with the interest that had accrued.

'I'm afraid I don't know how to do that,' she continued. 'May I ask you to wait a moment whilst I ring our main office to make some enquiries?'

Eagerly I waited, wondering how much my childhood efforts would now be worth. Five minutes later, she was back, looking a little sheepish. 'I'm afraid I must ask you for some photo ID,' she said.

I smiled; checks to safeguard against money laundering were obviously important, but I doubted that an international fraudster would be too interested in my thirteen shillings and sixpence!

I showed her my driving licence, and she compared my present signature with my effort as a twelve year-old. She then threw a bucket of cold water over my hopes and expectations.

'In 1969,' she explained, 'this form of savings was discontinued. Interest continued to be added to most accounts, but those with a balance of less than one pound were excluded. Therefore, I'm afraid the value of your savings remains 13 shillings and sixpence. Of course, decimalisation was introduced in 1971, so your 13 shillings and sixpence is now valued at 65p. Our central office has advised that I give it to you in the form of a stamp.'

Ruefully, I handed over my old book, and she formally closed the account. I asked her to return it to me as it was full of childhood memories. With a murmur of regret, she handed the book back to me together with a single first-class postage stamp.

***

Many more years were to pass before my son had his urgent need for a first-class stamp.

'Just wait here,' I said. 'I'll go and get one.'

I went to my study, unlocked the drawer in the desk where our passports, wills, and the deeds of the house were kept, and I retrieved the stamp.

'There you are, son,' I said. 'I've been saving this for a special occasion. I hope it brings you luck.'

A Misunderstanding and a Bully

'IT'S A BLOODY DISGRACE. YOU LOT COULDN'T ORGANISE A PISS UP IN THE PROVERBIAL BREWERY.' Geoff was busy dictating his notes on the old man he had just seen with a troublesome hernia when he heard the commotion coming from the waiting area just beyond the door.

'FOR GOD'S SAKE, GET THE MANAGER DOWN HERE TO SORT THINGS OUT.' He switched the dictating machine off for a moment to listen. He suspected the disturbance resulted from a patient's dissatisfaction at having to wait beyond the time of his appointment; not that this was an unusual event. Regrettably, it was par for the course when Mr Stephens was in the clinic; he frequently became so engrossed teaching the students that he completely lost track of time.

The consultant was an excellent teacher and enjoyed the company of the students, but unfortunately, the consequence of his enthusiasm was that as the morning progressed, patients waited longer and longer to be seen. By lunchtime, some poor patients might have been waiting for an hour or more.

The disturbance outside Geoff's room temporarily ceased and a moment later, his nursing assistant, Gladys Burrows, threw open the door. She confirmed Geoff's suspicions. It took a great deal to upset Gladys. For many years, she had worked as a nurse in the accident and emergency department. She was therefore accustomed to dealing with the drunks, drug addicts, and the diverse delinquents that disrupted the delivery of service in that department but she had not expected to witness such behaviour in the outpatient clinic. Her encounter with this patient had left her flustered.

'There's a patient outside called Colin Redman,' she reported, red-faced and angry. 'He's complained to me twice about the wait. He's upsetting the other patients, and making adverse comments to all and sundry, about the inefficiency of the Health Service in general, and about you in particular. He's the rudest man I've ever met, and I've met plenty of them in my time! His language is appalling. And there's a child in the waiting area as well. He complains he's been waiting for over an hour, but actually, that isn't true. One minute he says he's going to walk out of the hospital, the next he's threatening to write to the hospital manager. Worse, he's threatening that if you don't see him next; he'll come in here and knock your block off.'

It was already twelve-thirty, and Geoff wasn't feeling particularly sympathetic. He'd worked without a break since eight-thirty. His midmorning drink had been taken 'on the go' between patients, gulped down whilst recording one of the many consultations he had conducted. He had already seen fifteen or sixteen post-operative cases for their routine follow-up appointments. He'd checked their wounds, ensured there were no untoward complications and discharged them. In addition, there had been a number of new patients, including a child with an in growing toenail, another with a tight foreskin, and a couple of women with varicose veins.

Geoff was tempted to tell Nurse Burrows to give Mr Redman paper and pencil, so he could write to the Chief Executive, but he thought better of it; he would probably end up with an extra task, that of explaining the cause of the delay to the Complaints Manager. The line of least resistance, of course, was to expedite the man's consultation, but it was clearly inappropriate to reward rudeness and aggression, at the expense of those who were waiting patiently.

'How many patients have I got to see before him?'

'Just one, a twelve-year-old lad called Martin Bates; he's another lad with a foreskin problem. His GP seems to think he needs a circumcision. I doubt that it will take you too long to see him.'

'Then would you mind offering Mr Redman my apologies for the delay. Tell him that it's nearly his turn, but that it would be unfair to the young lad if he were to be seen first.'

Quite what was said in response to this message, Geoff never discovered but Gladys returned tight-lipped and grim-faced.

Geoff turned and spoke into the tannoy to call his next patient from the waiting area. 'Master Bates please, for room two.'

Ten seconds later, the door burst open, and Paul was confronted by another angry individual.

'I suppose you think that's funny.' Mrs Bates blazed, her son in tow behind her.

'You keep me waiting for three-quarters of an hour and then make fun of my boy.'

Geoff was nonplussed. He didn't understand her remark, nor did he comprehend why she should be angry. Even if she hadn't heard Nurse Burrows apologise to Mr Redman, surely she must have realised he had risked further alienating him by seeing her son first.

She should be grateful to him for resisting Mr Redman's pressure. Had he not done so, she would have waited even longer.

'I'm sorry,' he said, looking bemused. 'I know we've got behind schedule this morning, and I apologise for that; it's been a very busy clinic, but I don't understand how I've upset your lad.'

'Calling *Master Bates* like that over the loudspeaker. Don't you think he gets teased enough at school by the older boys? They don't realise the hurt they cause, but you.... a doctor......' In her anger, she left the sentence unfinished.

Suddenly, the penny dropped. *'Master Bates - masturbates'.* Geoff was horrified. It had been a totally innocent mistake, yet he immediately saw the upset he had caused, particularly if the boy was being bullied or victimised at school, simply because of his name.

'Look, I'm most awfully sorry,' he spluttered. 'I just didn't realise. I truly never even thought there could be a double meaning. Please forgive me.'

Mrs Bates looked daggers at him. 'Well, you really need to be more careful,' she stormed, 'particularly as he has this problem with his 'little Johnny'. He's a sensitive lad and easily gets upset.'

Geoff held up both hands. 'Look, all I can do is to apologise; I simply didn't realise.'

Martin's mother said nothing in response, and the consultation proceeded in an icy atmosphere.

In due course, Geoff explained to her the 'pros and cons' of a circumcision operation, before arranging for the lad's name to be added to the waiting list for surgery. He was relieved that she was so keen to get away from him that she didn't ask how long they would have to wait. He wouldn't have relished informing her the waiting time was likely to be between five and six months!

Then Geoff steeled himself in readiness to meet his next patient. As Mr Redman came through the door, Geoff said a polite *'Good morning'* and held out his hand. It was an old fashioned gesture, but something he did with all his patients. He felt it set an appropriate tone for the consultation. His hand was studiously ignored.

'I'm sorry that you've been kept waiting,' he said.

Mr Redman was not as Geoff had expected. He was a slightly-built, rather insignificant man, wearing a crumpled suit and scuffed shoes. But, true to his name, he was red in the face. He glared angrily at Geoff.

'I've been waiting over an hour and a half to see you,' he

stormed, waving his appointment card in Geoff's face. Then catching sight of the empty mug on the desk, he added, 'and I suppose you've just been sitting here, chatting with the nurses and drinking tea.'

Geoff controlled his own temper with difficulty. The clinic had undoubtedly been delayed, but there had been good reasons for that. In addition to Mr Stephens' enthusiasm for teaching, he had been called to resolve a problem on the ward, which had caused a ten-minute delay. Gladys Burrows had already said he'd been waiting for less than an hour, and she was now shaking her head vigorously from side to side, behind Mr Redman's back. Geoff decided to verify the time of the appointment to check Mr Redman's claim and hopefully to defuse his anger.

'May I see your appointment card, please?'

'Don't you believe me?' Mr Redman shouted.

Geoff was tempted to say '*no*' but he managed to control himself. 'Just to check, if you don't mind,' he said.

Reluctantly, Mr Redman released the card.

As Geoff had suspected, the patient should have been seen fifty minutes earlier, not an hour and a half earlier. 'I'm sorry we're behind schedule,' he said, 'but as I suspected, you haven't been waiting for 90 minutes, have you? In fact, it's less than an hour.'

'What if it is, it's still a damn disgrace. I'm a busy man. I haven't got time to waste sitting here twiddling my thumbs.'

Geoff was just about to hand the card back when he noticed the date on the top.

'What date is it today?' he asked Mr Redman, the suggestion of a smile on his face.

'Monday the first, of course.'

Geoff looked Mr Redman in the eye and held it for a moment before delivering what he felt sure would be the 'coup de gras'.

'Your appointment was for Monday, 1st of February. Today is Monday, 1st of March. You should have been here a month ago.'

For a moment, there was silence as Geoff returned the card.

'Well?' he asked, wondering whether Mr Redman would have the guts to apologise.

'Well, what of it?' he said bluntly, 'I'm here now, aren't I?

'Mr Redman, if you'd come, when you should have come, someone else could have had today's appointment, couldn't they?'

There was still no apology just a long silence before Mr Redman demanded, 'Well, are you going to deal with this lump on my arm, Doctor, or are you going to keep me waiting even longer?'

Geoff was staggered at this rudeness. Quickly he examined the lump, pronounced that it was an innocent fatty swelling, said that his name would be added to the waiting list, and within two minutes wished him a "*Good morning.*'

'Well, what did you make of that?' he asked Gladys, when Mr Redman had left.

'Quite unbelievable,' she responded. 'I suggest you put him at the very bottom of the waiting list, then when he comes in, get the clumsiest medical student you can find to operate on him. That's all he deserves!'

Geoff smiled. 'I could allow you to do his operation if you like,' he said, 'and provide you with a blunt and rusty scalpel to use as well.'

'That would be even better; something I should really enjoy!'

Thought for the day

I'll not listen to reason...Reason always means what someone else has to say.

Elizabeth Gaskell 1810 – 1865

'Is there a Doctor on Board?'

It's been an idyllic holiday. For the last fortnight, my wife and I have escaped the British winter and cruised around the Caribbean on a luxury liner. We've visited ten different islands; St Kitts, St Lucia, Dominica, and Martinique amongst them and, as I sit here on an Airbus 330 on the flight home, the long journey eased by the glass of Sauvignon Blanc I have in my hand, it's pleasant to reminisce about those green islands, blue skies, and warm seas. We're both determined to return and savour it all again at some stage in the future.

In my mind, I have a kaleidoscope of different memories. We've visited so many islands in such a short time that I now find it difficult to recall which of the many activities we enjoyed corresponded to each island; snorkelling on Guadeloupe, river tubing on Grenada (or was that on St Vincent) and yachting on Antigua, at least I think it was Antigua, though it might have been Grand Turk. They were all such beautiful islands, with lovely, friendly people. And all that music; happy music wherever we went, in the shops, on the coach trips and, of course, the calypso bands on the quayside whenever we boarded or left our floating hotel. Mind you; perhaps we did hear Bob Marley advising us 'Not to Worry' just a little too often. And we swam with huge stingrays too; we were able to stroke them – their skin was so smooth - almost like velvet. Now, where was that - perhaps it was St Vincent? And the weather in the Caribbean is perfect, isn't it? Warm and sunny, day after day, and should you feel a little too hot, you just go for a swim from one of those gorgeous, sandy beaches.

Life on board was effortless, our every need anticipated and catered for and the days slipped swiftly by. We usually went on deck at about eight in the morning, to watch the boat dock after its overnight journey from yesterday's island. How they manoeuvre a ship 300 yards long and weighing over 100,000 tons to glide so gently to the jetty is a miracle. Then breakfast; full English, if we were going ashore for some activity and planning to miss lunch; continental, if we intended to stay on board for the day.

Of course, everyone knows the food onboard is superb and there's so much of it! I confess we tried to be disciplined, but we've both managed to put on a pound or two. If you were so inclined, you could have a cooked breakfast, a midmorning snack of toast, crumpets, and teacakes, followed by a three-course lunch. Scones and cakes are available in the afternoon, and then, of course, a five-course, silver service meal in the evening. And if that's not enough food for you, the pizza and pancake bars are available until one in the morning. We didn't overindulge, but judging by the beached whales sunning themselves by the pool, plenty of others did.

Oops, hang on a minute! Here comes the air hostess again with a second glass of wine. I mustn't miss that! 'That's lovely, thanks very much.'

Since this was our first cruise, we didn't know which of the dining options to choose. One possibility was to opt for 'free dining' and simply go to any one of the many dining areas. You just turn up, as and when you choose and sit with whoever arrives at the same time. Alternatively, you can have 'fixed dining', sitting with the same people at the same table each evening. That's what we decided to do, and by and large, it worked well.

Inevitably, we got to know the other couples at our table well, and as always happens at the end of a holiday, we swopped contact details and promised to keep in touch - though if previous holidays are anything to go by, these commitments are unlikely to be fulfilled. On our table, there was a retired army general from Holland and his quiet little wife. I didn't know that Holland was a member of NATO until he told us about his involvement in joint exercises with our military. His wife was a little mouse who was difficult to engage in conversation, but they both spoke beautiful English; well, the continentals always do, don't they? It makes me rather ashamed of my education; I can just about get by in French, but I don't speak a word of Dutch.

Then there was a very interesting man who came from Watford; an engineer who'd spent his life designing bridges. His wife is a keen golfer, so she and my wife, Jane, got on well. The last couple came from Hereford, an accountant called Frank Purvis, and his wife, Mavis; both were pleasant enough, though Mavis was a bit intense and clingy. I thought she pried into our private life rather too much; Jane said she was just plain nosey! As it happens, they're on the same flight as us now, sitting a few rows behind.

When I'm on holiday, I don't like folk to know I'm a doctor. I don't have 'Doctor' recorded on my driving licence or passport, and

I don't go advertising the fact when in the company of strangers. If your medical background slips out, it seems the whole world and his dog feel entitled to a free opinion on their various illnesses, the problems of their friends and relatives, and on occasions, even of their pets. People seem to think you will be interested in all their previous illnesses as well; the time they fell off a camel in Egypt and fractured their collar bone, or the occasion when their son got prickly heat when he was camping and the scoutmaster brought everyone home because he thought it was measles.

I've even had a woman regale me with the gory details of her prolapse operation. I have a son who is a physio and a daughter who is a dietician, and I know the same thing happens to them. Imagine what it must be like for midwives if every woman they meet insists on regaling them with all the intimate details of their time in labour. Fortunately, I'm able to tell them that my knowledge of their various problems could be written on the back of a postcard; you see I'm a retired psychiatrist, and when they learn that, they usually shut up. There shouldn't be a stigma about mental health, though unfortunately there still is, and people rarely admit to being sufferers.

My reverie is interrupted by an announcement.

'Good evening, this is your captain speaking. I'm sorry that we were a little late leaving Barbados. This was due to the late arrival of the incoming flight, which encountered a headwind of 120 mph. However, that same wind will speed our return journey, so we should be able to make up most of the time. Our expected flight time is eight hours and twenty minutes.

Shortly, the cabin staff will come through the cabin and serve you with your evening meal. Then the lights will be dimmed to allow you a chance to sleep. So please, settle down, enjoy the flight, and I will speak to you again shortly before we arrive at Gatwick.'

I suppose airlines do their best to make passengers feel comfortable, but eight hours in a cramped space, eating plastic food from a plastic tray is not my idea of heaven - but I guess it's the price we must pay when travelling long distances to reach fabulous locations. I find the only way to cope is simply to do as you are told and go with the flow; do this, do that, queue here, wait there - all the while, trying to be patient and phlegmatic.

I've eaten my meal, it was only a small portion but quite tasty. I've had a coffee and finished that second glass of wine. The lights are low. I've a mask over my eyes, and I'm searching for sleep when I hear another announcement over the tannoy, muted by the plugs I'm wearing in my ears.

'If there is a doctor on board, will they please make themselves known to a member of the cabin crew?'

I groan and sink further into my seat. It's the one thing I dread when travelling.

There are nearly three hundred people on the plane; surely, I'm not the only doctor on board. I'll close my eyes, pretend to be asleep, then wait and hope that someone else answers the call.

Then I hear a voice behind me calling for the steward, and surreptitiously I look over my shoulder. Mrs Purvis, busybody that she is, is talking to the steward and pointing in my direction. Privately, I curse her.

The steward is speaking to me now. 'I wonder if I can have a word with you, Sir. I understand that you're a doctor. I'm afraid we have a passenger who requires urgent medical assistance. Perhaps you could follow me?'

He doesn't offer me any choice, I note, though I guess he's right – I don't really have any choice!

He leads me towards the front of the plane, past the toilets, through the forward section, then on towards the front exit doors. All eyes are upon me as I trail behind the steward. We go behind the screen to the area where the cabin crew prepare the meals. I am amazed to see how cramped it is.

Lying on the floor is an elderly man. He is semi-conscious.

My heart sinks. I haven't a clue where to begin.

'Look,' I say desperately, 'I'm just not qualified to deal with this. I was a psychiatrist, but I've been retired for more than ten years.'

'But it seems you're the only doctor on board,' the steward says, 'and obviously that makes you better qualified than we are.'

I remember that I no longer hold any indemnity against claims of medical negligence, but vaguely recall reading somewhere that Good Samaritan acts usually escape litigation.

'We have a defibrillator on board,' the steward continues, 'I'll go and get it.'

I look again at the man on the floor. Clearly, I have no choice but to see what I can do, despite the fact that its forty years since I last practised any physical medicine.

Although semiconscious, he has a reasonable colour. I kneel at his side and feel for his pulse. At least I know how to do that! To give myself some thinking time, I measure it over thirty seconds, but even then, I can't think what to do next.

The steward returns with the defibrillator and takes it out of its case. I've never seen one before! It strikes me the steward will have had some first-aid training. If we have to use it, at least he will know how it works because I certainly don't!

'Hopefully we're not going to need that,' I say out loud, though mainly I suspect for my own reassurance.

I feel the panic rising in my chest, and my mind becomes a blur. I'm conscious of the steward standing over me, expecting me to be competent and professional when I know that any boy scout with his first-aid badge would have a better idea of what to do.

Now the man on the floor is attempting to speak, and I try to make out what he's saying. One word is clear enough to understand....'diabetic'.

My God, I think; what the hell do I remember about diabetes. Finally, one constructive thought penetrates my befuddled mind. If he's diabetic, he'll be travelling with some tablets or insulin.

'Is he travelling alone?' I ask.

'Yes, he is.'

'Does he have a bag or any hand-luggage with him? Perhaps there will be something there that may help us.'

He returns with the man's case, and we rifle through it. Sure enough, there's a supply of insulin, and a collection of needles and syringes.

So, he is indeed diabetic. But now I'm more concerned than before, and even more aware of my own inadequacies. Is his present condition due to his diabetes, or is diabetes just a red herring and he's actually suffering from some unrelated problem, possible a heart attack? And if this is a diabetic coma, is this due to a low blood sugar or a high one?

I honestly haven't a clue how to distinguish high from low, and if I assume it's a high blood sugar, give him a shot of insulin and it turns out he's got a low blood sugar, I shall probably kill him. And the steward is still standing over me, observing my every move, expecting me to know what to do.

A stewardess arrives and piles more pressure on me.

'The captain urgently needs your assessment of the situation,' she says. 'We're mid-Atlantic, and he has to decide whether to continue to London or divert to Tenerife.' As if I haven't already got enough on my plate!

'Well, to tell you the truth,' I start to admit, 'I really don't....' and then the most marvellous thing happens.

The screen is pulled back and a tall good-looking man of about forty strolls through.

'I hear you have a bit of medical problem,' he says, his voice oozing confidence. 'I would have come sooner, but I was asleep.'

'Are you a doctor?' I ask, praying that he is.

'Yes,' he says, 'I'm a consultant in Emergency Medicine,' he adds and mentions one of the largest and most prestigious hospitals in London.

'Thank God, I'm so relieved to meet you,' I reply. 'I'm sure you are much better qualified to deal with this problem than this elderly retired psychiatrist.'

Hugely relieved, I return to my seat.

Mrs Purvis immediately rushes to speak with me. 'What was the problem? It must be so exciting for you; so wonderful that you're able to help in an emergency like this. What a tale I shall have to tell my friends when I get home! Is the patient all right?'

'Yes,' I say, as cool as you like. 'It was really no problem at all; everything's now safely under control so, if you will excuse me, it's time for me to get back to sleep.'

Thought for the day

Any man who goes to a psychiatrist should have his head examined.

Sam Goldwyn 1882 – 1974

The Dietician's Tale

My patient came through the door, waddled into the room, then slowly, and with a sigh, eased himself into the chair. It groaned under his weight, and I feared for its safety. One look at him told me he was obese, but the protocol insisted that I had to calculate his Body Mass Index, and chart it for his records. The measurement, whatever it proved to be, would be the base-line against which his efforts at weight loss, and my success as a dietician would be measured.

'Let's have you on the scales,' I said without much enthusiasm. Some inner instinct told me that this man had little interest in reducing his weight. The chair groaned again as he levered himself to his feet. He struggled to the scales. He weighed 101 kilograms (15st 12lbs). By this time, he was slightly short of breath, so I gave him a moment to recover before asking him to stand against the wall to be measured. He was 1.67 metres tall (5 ft 6 ins). I plotted the readings on the conversion chart; his BMI was 36! That made the diagnosis of 'obesity' official!

I settled myself down and picked up a weight-reduction leaflet. It was the last in the folder, so I made a mental note to order some more. I see hundreds of overweight patients every year. It's by far the commonest condition I have to treat, and I confess it takes quite an effort to sound spontaneous and enthusiastic when repeating the same advice over and over again. However, his health and life expectancy would be greatly enhanced if he could be persuaded to lose weight, so I determined to do my best; I would give it my best shot.

I started by warning him of all the dangers of obesity; high-blood-pressure and strokes, diabetes, heart attacks, arthritis, and so on. I always lay considerable emphasis on the fact that all these conditions can lead to an earlier death, thus emphasising their importance. He listened politely, though without showing a great deal of interest. Then we discussed the many ways in which his obesity affected his day to day lifestyle; his reduced mobility, his breathlessness and the wear and tear on the joints in his feet, legs, hips, and spine. This seemed to claim his attention a little more.

'Are you saying that if I lose weight, my knees won't trouble me as much,' he asked.

'That's exactly what I'm saying,' I replied. 'With every step you take, your entire body weight is carried on your knees; and not only on your knees but on your hips and ankles as well. Obviously, with less weight to carry, your legs will trouble you less. You will be less breathless as well.'

The fact that he was now showing a little more interest encouraged me to up my game.

'There are so many ways to lose weight,' I enthused, 'and so many programmes available to help you along the way.'

Most dieticians I know, at this point in the consultation, start to talk about dieting. Clearly, this is important, but my view is that dieting is usually seen in a negative light by patients. They often have preconceived ideas of being obliged to give up the sweets, crisps, and cakes they enjoy, in favour of lettuce leaves and carrots! My own preference is to begin by enquiring what activities or hobbies the patient enjoys, or has enjoyed in the past, such as walking, swimming or cycling, to see whether these can be encouraged. I also like to stress that their body-image and self-confidence will be improved if they can shed those rolls of fat.

On this occasion, I found my patient had been football-mad as a youngster, and I was able to inform him of a programme of walking football that had recently been introduced at the local gym. Now, I felt I had him; he was enthusiastic and motivated. Perhaps my earlier negativity had been misplaced; maybe I might have success with this patient after all.

Inevitably, I moved on to discuss his diet. As expected, it was not a healthy one. Chocolate cereals, buttered toast and marmalade washed down with sweet tea at breakfast, a couple of Mars bars and crisps for lunch, then sausage or fried fish with chips for his evening meal. By this time, however, the consultation was going well. I had my patient's attention; he was positive, motivated and enthusiastic. He declared he would give his all to the diet and exercise regime I'd prescribed for him.

Pleased with the way things had gone, I wished him luck and arranged a follow-up appointment for him. Then I gave myself a well-earned pat on the back; I'd gee'ed myself up at the start of the consultation and it was going to pay dividends.

'Thanks so much for your help. I'll see you in two months then,' he said as he left. 'I shall have lost two stones by then.'

'That would be great,' I said, though I knew that even for a determined individual, this would be a tall order. 'Particularly remember that processed foods and sugary drinks are to be avoided. There are ten teaspoons of sugar in every can of Coke.' I added as a parting shot.

'I will, I will,' he assured me.

***

Actually, I didn't have to wait two months to see him again. We saw each other at McDonalds during lunch. He had a Big Mac burger, French fries and a large Coke in front of him, and as it happened, so did I!

One Leg or Two?

Jim was convalescing in a side ward on the vascular unit of a well-known London hospital after an emergency operation to repair a ruptured abdominal aortic aneurysm. Four days early, he had never heard of the condition. The major artery that carries all the blood to the lower half of his body, a motorway of a vessel half an inch wide, had suffered a 'blow out' such as may occur on a car tyre. The 'blow out' had then burst. The ward sister had said that the majority of people, who experience such a devastating event, don't live to tell the tale! They die of blood loss, usually before they even reach the hospital.

Fortunately, the operation had been a success, the bleeding had been arrested and Jim had been dragged back from the Pearly Gates. Blood was now flowing smoothly into his legs, through the artificial tube the surgeons had used to replace the burst blood vessel.

Jim had been allocated a side room whilst he had been so ill, but was now able to wander onto the main ward during the day. Being a sociable fellow, he had not enjoyed the isolation of his single room, and was now chatting with Cliff who had just been admitted.

'The doctors tell me that smoking is the main reason my blood vessel burst,' Jim remarked when asked about his problems. 'I've been a *'twenty-a-day man'* all my life. I started smoking when I was in the army; well you could buy cigarettes so cheaply in the forces, couldn't you? But I guess I'll have to give it up now otherwise I'll get more trouble.'

'Giving smoking up isn't so easy, you know,' Cliff responded. 'I was given the same advice a couple of years ago when I lost my leg.' He nodded to the artificial limb that was propped up at the bedside. 'But I couldn't do it. Now the arteries in my other leg are clogged up. The damn thing's going gangrenous just like the first one did. I've watched my toes slowly going purple, and now they're black. For weeks, I've been hoping for the best but fearing the worst. The pain is terrible, it's giving me hell. That's why I've come in. The doctors say they can do nothing to save it, so it's coming off this afternoon. At least that will get rid of the pain, but God only knows how I'll manage with no legs.'

As they continued to chat, Cliff's family arrived to support him and wish him luck, so Jim moved on to talk with the other patients, hoping they had more cheerful tales to tell.

For the first few hours after his operation, Cliff was closely monitored and heavily sedated. During the night, however, he became restless and extremely confused. He shouted, thrashed around in his bed, and several times tried to climb out, despite the cot sides that the nurses had provided. The noise and disturbance was such that no one on the ward could get any sleep, so shortly after midnight Jim was asked to swop beds with Cliff who was moved into the side room.

Regrettably, Cliff's condition continued to deteriorate and at three in the morning, he collapsed. The emergency medical team rushed to the scene and the Night Sister, fearing the worst, called the relatives. Breathless and anxious they arrived on the ward, dashed to the bed where they expected Cliff to be and pulled back the screens, waking Jim as they did so.

'My god,' Jim heard Cliff's wife exclaim, 'they've not taken his other leg off – they've stitched the first one back on again!'

(Based on a story by Mr G Leigh-Ford)

The Hazards of Falling in Love

It seems to me in these modern times, that when a young man invites a girl out for a meal or suggests they go to the cinema or to a party, he expects her to be stork-proof, and willing to stay for breakfast. But in the days before the pill, free love and flower power, things were very different. Courting, or 'walking out' as it was sometimes referred to, was a sedate affair; relationships progressing far more slowly than is the case today.

Furthermore, parents oversaw any developing romance closely, not wanting their offspring to waste their lives with an unsuitable partner. In particular, they felt especially protective towards any daughter they might have, dreading that she might get into trouble (or 'into the family way' as folk used to say). In those days, parents became concerned if the amorous couple occupied their living room late into the evening. What were they up to? Was it safe for them to retire to bed, whilst the boyfriend was on the settee cuddling their daughter? Father might well go downstairs on some pretence, perhaps to get a glass of milk, supposedly to ease his heartburn, just to keep an eye on things. Such old-fashioned attitudes of parents were certainly justified when there were young men like Brian roaming the neighbourhood.

Brian was a good-looking, easy-going, 28-year-old Lothario, who left a trail of broken hearts wherever he went. By no means unintelligent, (he left school at the age of 18, having obtained good grades in his 'A' level exams), he decided to take a break before going to university. He travelled the world, foot-loose and fancy-free, enjoying himself enormously, only undertaking casual work as and when his funds ran low. This 'gap' year became two years, and then three. Returning to the UK, he continued to drift, gambling occasionally, drinking frequently, until a suspended sentence for a drugs offence and a stern lecture from the local magistrate, forced him to reconsider his lifestyle. He concluded it was time for him to settle down and decided he would like to study medicine. Allowing his creative imagination free rein when filling in his application form, (bodyboarding on Bondi Beach became missionary work in Malaysia), he was accepted as a mature student at a Medical School in London.

It transpired that the term *mature*, whilst accurate in respect of his age relative to the other students, was distinctly inaccurate in terms of his behaviour. Brian struggled to reform his lifestyle, finding it impossible to give appropriate attention to the lectures and tutorials of his degree course, whilst drinking and partying with his friends. The result was that he failed several exams and was dropped down a year. Twice, he was hauled before the Dean of his Medical School, Professor Hambleton, and formally reprimanded. On the first occasion, the Dean lectured him severely for failing to apply himself to his studies, but on the second, after a fracas in the city centre which came to the attention of the police, the warning was brutal and final.

'This is your last chance,' the Dean declared, 'one more misdemeanour, no matter how insignificant, and I shall expel you; in which case you will never qualify as a doctor. Is that absolutely clear?'

They say that opposites attract, and Brian's life was turned upside down when he met Mary at a Medical School dance. Ten years his junior, she was the sweetest, nicest young nurse that anyone could hope to meet. The only child of a professional couple, she had led a carefully sheltered life, attending a good Catholic girl's boarding school, and undertaking voluntary work in a local care home in her school holidays. Her mother was a nursing sister in the local hospice, and it had come as no surprise when Mary had announced that she too wished to become a nurse.

The moment Mary met Brian she was smitten. He was handsome, confident, widely-travelled and good company. With his 'easy come, easy go' attitude, he was unlike anyone else she had ever met. Inevitably, her friends warned her of his reputation, but Brian was showing her that life could be fun, so she paid them no heed. She was, however, aware that her parents might not approve, so she failed to mention her boyfriend on her periodic visits home. As the friendship developed into a relationship, Mary's parents became increasingly inquisitive about her frequent 'weekends away with friends', so Mary felt obliged to tell them about Brian. In truth, she was so much in love with him that she was actually bursting to show him off.

Inevitably, her parents were keen to meet Brian, to judge him for themselves but, conscious that her father was a particularly stern and formidable man, Mary decided it would be best if Brian should meet her mother first. Accordingly, she arranged that the meeting should take place when her father was away from home.

The meeting was a disaster from the very start.

'Your face seems familiar to me, have we met somewhere before?' Brian asked, the minute he arrived.

'Yes', Mary's mother replied sternly. 'We met this morning, on the tube. You were sitting and I was standing - all the way from Liverpool Street to Leytonstone.'

It took her less than twenty minutes, to get the measure of the man who had won her daughter's heart, and after Brian had departed, she made her views known to Mary in a forthright fashion.

The bond of love that binds two people together, however, can be strong. Mary was in love with Brian, she was in love with the life he had shown her and the newfound freedom she was enjoying. As a result, her mother's words went unheeded. The relationship continued, Brian having no further contact with Mary's parents until the inevitable happened; Mary became pregnant.

Brian was not altogether without scruples and agreed that they should get married. A secret runaway Gretna Green marriage was discussed, but reluctantly Brian agreed with Mary, that her parents should be told.

'Do you think your Dad will have much to say when I tell him we're going to get married?' Brian asked.

'I don't know,' Mary replied, 'But since I'm pregnant, he certainly would if you told him we weren't!'

For any young man who has serious intentions towards his beloved, there has always been the apprehension of that terrifying first meeting with the girl's father. Whilst Brian was hoping to be accepted into Mary's family, after the trauma of his meeting with her mother, he was fearful at the thought of facing her father. For days before the meeting, he agonised about what he should wear and what he should say, hoping to be accepted, but afraid of his anger and rejection.

Apprehensively, Mary at his side, they opened the front door. Mary's father stood before them. Brian's heart sank; it was Professor Hambleton, the Dean of the Medical School!

'So, it's you,' he growled. 'Damn you! I said I'd throw you out if you got into trouble again. Now that you've got my daughter into trouble, I suppose I shall have to let you qualify as a doctor so that you'll be able to support her!'

Mary's parents arranged a quiet wedding a few weeks later, with only their immediate family and closest friends invited. However, many of Brian's friends attended the church service, one of them acting as an usher showing people to their seats.

'Are you a friend of the bridegroom?' he asked politely of one particularly stern lady at the church door.

'No, I certainly am not,' came the grim reply, 'I'm the bride's mother.'

This tale is based on some observations of courting by John Aye whose humorous thoughts on a variety of subjects are well worth reading.

Thought for the day

To keep your marriage brimming
With love in the loving cup
Whenever you're wrong, admit it
Whenever you're right. Shut up!
Ogden Nash 1902 - 1971

The Vegetable Marrow

'Now, before you go, I have a favour to ask of you.'

Inwardly Paul groaned; yet more jobs to be heaped on their shoulders. Surely their lives as junior doctors were hectic enough without performing 'favours' for their consultant?

'As I think you know,' Sir William explained, 'I'm a keen gardener. I enjoy growing vegetables in my spare time, not just to eat but also to enter in local competitions. The hospital's summer fete is being held in a couple of weeks, and I need someone to keep an eye on my marrows for me.'

Treating his patients was all very well, they got paid for that, but caring for his vegetables as well? That was beyond the pale. But they were in no position to argue, they depended on him for a reference. Cross him and their prospects of promotion might suddenly fall.

'I've won prizes twice in the last three years,' Sir William enthused, 'and I'd love to make it a hat trick of wins. The care given to marrows in the final days before a show is critical but, unfortunately, I've some college business in London to attend to, and I'll be away for the next two weekends. Sadly, this year my marrows aren't as large or healthy as usual. We've had rather a cool summer and they need a bit of intensive care, ideally a settled spell of warm weather. I'd be grateful if you could keep an eye on them when I'm away.'

The task didn't sound too onerous; indeed it might even prove a welcome diversion from their work on the wards, so Saeed and Paul agreed to help, not that it would have been politic to do anything else! As far as housemen are concerned – whatever the consultant wants – the consultant gets! His slightest wish is their command!

Sir William went on to describe the attention the marrows required, and later gave them detailed written instructions on their feeding and watering. The time and care he gave to his marrows was obviously every bit as important to him as the time and care he lavished on his patients. The two junior doctors assured him that they would be extremely attentive and that he had no reason to be concerned.

The following Saturday afternoon, Saeed and Paul went to Sir

William's garden to inspect the vegetable marrows and see if they required any attention. His house had originally been the lodge to an old hall which had long since been demolished to make room for the hospital. It adjoined one of the city's municipal parks but was separated from it by a high fence, presumably to protect it from the local youths. The garden, amounting roughly to half an acre and was immaculately maintained; it was clearly the consultant's pride and joy. Walking around the side of the house, they found themselves on a small, covered veranda boasting an old bamboo easy chair, surrounded by tubs and troughs overflowing with late summer colour.

They presumed Sir William sat and rested here, admiring his handiwork, when his day's work was done. A gravel path led down the garden with a closely-mown lawn to one side, beyond which were mature apple and pear trees coming into fruit. Within the lawn was a circular bed full of magnificent roses in full bloom, no doubt the source of the buttonholes Sir William liked to wear on his jackets. On the other side of the path, was a well-maintained herbaceous border, again ablaze with colour. Dianthus, oxalis, and lavender occupied the front of the border. Behind them, achillea, dahlias and chrysanthemums jostled for space with the delphiniums. Further back, shrubs such as fuchsias, maples, and spirea added different textures and extra colour.

Beyond the lawn and flower bed, and furthest from the house, was the vegetable plot, and it was clear that this was where the consultant devoted his greatest efforts. Parts were free of plants, the early summer vegetables, such as broad beans and spring onions having been harvested, but even these areas had already been covered in compost to prepare the ground for the following season. Other areas held the mid-season and autumn crops such as peas, carrots, dwarf and runner beans, and these were still being harvested. All looked strong and healthy without a weed to be seen between the various rows. Paul took the liberty of plucking a pod of peas to nibble; then helped himself to a few more, as they tasted so good.

'You'd better take those empty pods back to the residency or hide them in the compost heap,' Saeed advised, 'to remove all evidence of your crime.'

At the far end of the plot, the turnips, sprouts and swedes were waiting to be cropped through the winter.

In pride of place, in the sunniest part of the vegetable garden, were the marrows. There were three of them, and it was difficult to decide which had pride of place. They were about four feet long and so wide that it would have been difficult to encircle them with both arms. Light green in colour, with broader stripes of a richer, darker green along their length, they rested on purpose-built net hammocks which held them off the ground to protect them from slugs, and to prevent any soiling or discolouration of their skins from contact with the ground. The elasticated material from which the hammocks were made bore a remarkable resemblance to the elastic hosiery used by patients after operations on their varicose veins!

Sir William had given them written instructions, typed no doubt by his hospital secretary, detailing exactly how the marrows had to be watered and fed. There were two different feeds; a granular fertiliser to be spread around the roots, and a liquid one that apparently contained the trace elements necessary to remedy any deficiencies in the soil.

'It's like dispensing vitamins and tonics to our malnourished patients on the ward,' Paul said, 'except these are by no means frail specimens; they're bursting with health.'

Saeed glanced at the giant marrows, barely restrained by the supporting netting. 'More like giving performance enhancing drugs to weightlifters, I would have thought!' he observed.

They had also been instructed to look for any evidence of slug activity, to lay slug pellets if necessary and to check that the hammocks were giving adequate support. Apparently, it was important to carry the weight of the marrows to prevent any undue stretching of the stalk. Dutifully they fulfilled these tasks.

It was impossible not to admire the size, colour and texture of such magnificent specimens. They certainly impressed Saeed.

'They're fantastic, he said, 'I've absolutely no doubt they will win First Prize at the hospital's summer fete.'

'I'm not so sure,' Paul replied, 'I've been to one or two of these fruit and vegetable shows, and some of the exhibits are quite amazing. I've seen carrots two feet long and perfectly symmetrical. Gardeners grow them in large plastic drainpipes in a mixture of sand, compost, and nutrients. I have seen leeks as thick as a man's arm, cauliflowers as big as footballs, and, on occasion, I've seen marrows larger than these.'

At first, Saeed was disinclined to believe this but Paul assured him that it was true.

'Then in that case, I think we should give these marrows a helping hand,' he said.

'Meaning?' Paul asked.

'Well, we could select one of them, perhaps this marrow in the centre is the pick of the bunch, then drip feed it for 24 hours. If we infuse it with two or three litres of saline, we could really plump it up. We're not overlooked here, so no-one will know. The fence and potting shed protects us from being seen by anyone in the park and we can't be seen from the hospital because of the house.'

'I'm not sure that's wise,' Paul said. 'Sir William has old fashioned values, I don't think he would approve'.

'I'm certain that he wouldn't. He wouldn't dream of doing anything underhand. But you know how badly he wants to win and he's not going to find out, is he?'

Paul felt anxious and had a premonition that something might go wrong. Perhaps the infused fluid would drip back out of the puncture wound, making the interference obvious, or worse, they might even kill the marrow. But Saeed's mind was made up.

'Come on,' he said, 'we need to get a few bits of equipment.'

The two junior doctors slipped back to the ward, returning with a drip stand, a delivery set, a long needle, and three large bags, each containing a litre of saline. Saeed carefully inserted the needle into the marrow just at the point where the stalk was attached so that it wouldn't be visible. Paul rigged up the drip stand, delivery set and first bag of saline. The drip worked beautifully and the bag was empty within a few minutes although it produced no visible change in the outward appearance of the marrow. The infusion slowed when they put up the second bag although there was still no obvious change in the marrow's size. Saeed suggested that it might take a little time for the skin to stretch and said he would return later to infuse the third bag.

The next day, Paul wasn't free to accompany Saeed to review the situation in Sir William's vegetable plot. He was busy attending to some new admissions on the ward, but Saeed reported all was well, and that the marrow they had infused looked plumper and healthier than before. They agreed they should return in seven days' time, to see if a further infusion was necessary.

The following Saturday, having confirmed that Sir William had indeed gone to London, they went to review the marrow they had doctored. It was gratifying to observe that, thanks to their administrations, it had grown considerably both in length and breadth during the previous seven days. Indeed, with its extra weight, it now almost touched the ground despite the support from the hammock. They noticed that, since their last visit, Sir William had placed straw underneath it, for added protection. Paul's concern that the saline might have killed the marrow was clearly unfounded; the marrow's skin appeared to have ripened, and the slight wrinkles that had existed previously had filled and disappeared. They also felt that the marrow's colour had improved with a greater distinction between the darker and the lighter green stripes that passed along its length. Their efforts as vegetable doctors were clearly being successful and they spent a little time congratulating each other.

They fed and watered all three marrows as before and, following their instructions, again placed slug pellets around their stems and adjusted the hammocks to take the strain off the stalks. Saeed walked around the marrow in the centre, and looked at it critically from all sides. Thanks to the infusion they had administered, it now outshone its neighbours. It was clearly the one Sir William would choose as his entry for the show.

'I think,' he said, after some deliberation and with the confidence that comes from complete ignorance of growing vegetables, 'that it would benefit from a further infusion.'

Again, Paul had doubts and pointed out that they didn't want the marrow to win by such a margin that people became suspicious. However, Saeed, as before, was adamant, so they returned to the ward and gathered together the equipment just as they had the previous weekend. This time, however, there was a problem. Perhaps not surprisingly, the stocks of saline in the storeroom were low, and there was a danger that if they depleted them further, none would be available should a patient need it.

'The nurses are a bit slow replenishing their supplies,' Saeed commented, with pretence at innocence, 'I think you'd better have a word with our ward sister, Paul.'

To avoid reducing the stocks further, they took three big bags of dextrose sugar solution as an alternative.

'This will be even better than saline,' Saeed remarked. 'Dextrose is pure carbohydrate, marrows are full of sugar, so this should work a treat. These extra bags will guarantee that Sir William wins his coveted first prize.'

They set up the drip as before and ensured that it was running freely. Saeed agreed to come back later to change the bags, and then return on the Sunday to review the situation before their boss returned. At that final visit, he would return the equipment to the ward and remove any evidence that the marrow had been given a helping hand.

***

The day of the garden fete was blessed with glorious weather; there wasn't a cloud in the sky, and the temperature rose by mid-afternoon to 80 degrees. Tied to the ward, thanks to the responsibility for his patients, Paul only heard later about the dramatic events that were to become a part of the hospital's folk lore.

Shortly after lunch, Sir William asked for Saeed's help to take the marrow from his garden to the marquee in the park where the entries for the different categories of vegetable were to be displayed and judged. Working slowly and gently, they cut the stalk, lifted the marrow from its hammock and placed it carefully on old cushions in a large wheelbarrow. It was so heavy that the two of them needed their combined strength to lift it. Taking great care to avoid any bumps in the path, the marrow was wheeled to the competition tent in the show ground, labelled and placed on the trestle table that had been allocated for the marrows, cucumbers and pumpkins. Saeed then felt obliged to wander round the show with Sir William, whilst waiting for the judging to take place. The hospital consultant was known to almost everyone there, and stopped frequently to chat with his colleagues, friends, and acquaintances. They all enquired about his marrows, and offered him their best wishes for another successful day.

After a while, Saeed excused himself and visited the various stalls and amusements. He threw cloth balls at plastic ducks, fished for prizes in the Lucky Wishing Well and took a turn on the Bottle Tom-bola. Later, he joined a group of nurses who, like him, were in need of a drink on such a warm day and escorted them to the beer tent for some liquid refreshment. Staying for an hour or so until late in the afternoon, he heard the announcement that the judges had completed their work and that the prize giving ceremony was about to commence. He finished his drink and then, eager to see if the nefarious assistance they had rendered the marrow would reap its unjust reward, he drifted back to the competition tent.

The heat in the marquee was stifling, but Saeed was delighted to see that Sir William's marrow was larger than the others by a considerable margin; indeed it dwarfed the other entries. Furthermore, whereas its rivals had deep wrinkles in their skins, Sir William marrow had a shining glossy coat; it appeared to be in the very best of health. It was certainly a magnificent specimen, and Saeed was in no doubt there could only be one winner. Surely, it would not only win the prize for best marrow, but also the prestigious 'Best in Entire Show' award.

Judging of the root vegetables had been completed and the results for the peas and beans were being announced as Saeed joined Sir William amongst the expectant crowd waiting to see if the father figure of the hospital would once again win first prize for his marrow. The judging of the marrows was to be the grand finale of the show, and there was great excitement as the chief judge moved, microphone in hand, to the tables upon which the cucumbers, pumpkins and marrows were displayed. He announced the first, second and third prizes for the cucumbers, each announcement being greeted with polite applause.

He then moved to the pumpkin table and was announcing the first prize when a short, but loud rasping sound, interrupted him; it was as if somebody had inadvertently passed flatus. The judge stopped mid-sentence but, since all now seemed quiet, he continued. The winner of the pumpkin prize stepped forward to receive a rosette from the judge, who went on to announce the second and third place winners of the pumpkin competition. However, whilst doing so, he was interrupted two or three times by much louder, longer, and this time moister sounds, which seemed to be coming from the marrow table. He looked anxiously at the marrows but spotted nothing amiss.

Finally, as he moved to the marrow table, the noise returned; louder, wetter and now continuous. All eyes in the crowd turned to search for its source, a source that was now all too apparent. A mixture of foul yellow liquid and gas was belching from the base of Sir William's marrow. A patient with dysentery could not have performed better. Further, as the discharge continued, the marrow was visibly shrinking, its skin crinkling and collapsing. The judge and audience watched the spectacle with a mixture of amazement and horror. Handkerchiefs were held to noses as the marrow continued to writhe, shrivel and shrink until it was nothing more than an empty green sack in a sea of offensive yellow fluid. A foul stench filled the air.

There was a mixed reaction from the audience. Initially, there was a gasp of surprise from the assembled throng, but, unfortunately, someone started to laugh and soon the entire crowd was in stitches, roaring with laughter. Saeed was horrified, he dared not look in Sir William's direction, but knew that he must be appalled and humiliated, since everyone knew to whom this particular marrow belonged.

The judge proved to be a quick-thinking man with a cool head. Unfazed by the spectacle unfolding before him, he didn't lose his composure. Whilst waiting for the crowd to quieten, he had to call for silence at least twice, he calmly slipped the card that had been on the top of the pack in his hand to the bottom. He laid his hand on the marrow that had been the second largest and announced that this had won the first prize. He subsequently gave the second prize to the marrow that would have been third.

'There will be no third prize for marrows this year' he announced.

A Hermit's Demise

Inevitably, the emotions that funerals evoke vary greatly, depending on the relationship that one has had with the deceased. The death of a child or young adult, a life cut short, its promise unfulfilled, is incredibly sad and a profound challenge for those with faith. In contrast, when an individual dies who has achieved great things in a long and fruitful life, be that in a public capacity or in the privacy of a family setting, the funeral and wake can truly be a celebration of a life well-lived, as was the case when my brother died recently.

In his seventieth year, my brother developed an abdominal tumour, which he knew would be incurable. He faced his illness with admirable courage. His life had mainly been spent in the hospitality field, as a chef and hotelier, but he had enthusiastically pursued a wide variety of other interests and, as a result, had a great many friends from different backgrounds. He delighted in cooking wholesome meals for his friends and his weekly 'suppers' were joyful occasions and greatly appreciated.

It was, therefore, no surprise that there was a full house for his funeral, which though intensely sad for his immediate family and the closest of his friends, was a surprisingly cheerful affair. In advance, he had personally planned the church service and the wake, and his wishes were followed to the letter. He had requested a wonderful selection of food and drink for his 'guests' and those present enjoyed an unforgettable feast in his memory.

Sadly the funerals of the very elderly are often quite different, especially of those who have outlived their siblings, their school or college friends and their old workmates. They may have spent their eightieth or ninetieth years living alone, possibly in a care home, and sometimes their funeral may be attended by a solitary neighbour and the funeral director. The following tale, which comes from Canada, tells of one such case.

One Sunday morning, Mason Woodall, who had set out for a day's fishing, found Owen Anderson collapsed and unconscious at the side of a country road in the backwoods of Nova Scotia. Mason was a care worker and occasional musician. From time to time, he played the bagpipes at local gigs and was always in demand each year for Burn's night suppers on the 25th January.

At first, Mason thought that Owen was dead, but on closer examination, he noted shallow, laboured breathing, and he found a weak pulse. His first thought was to call for the air ambulance but quickly decided that in the time it would take for the helicopter to arrive, he could drive the 40 miles to Caledonia where medical help was available. Gently, he lifted Owen onto the back seat of his pickup truck, secured him as best he could with the seat belts and set off at great speed. He was relieved that Owen survived the journey, and gratefully handed his care to the hospital staff. He presumed that would be the end of his involvement with Owen, but as it turned out, it wasn't.

In the hospital, it was found that Owen was hypothermic and had pneumonia. When he was warmed and his chest infection treated with antibiotics, he regained consciousness, but regrettably, further investigations revealed an underlying cancer of the lung, which was beyond cure. Accordingly, he was transferred to a local care home where it chanced that Mason, his roadside saviour, was employed.

Owen lived in the home for two months before he died, and during that time, the staff got to know him well. He was 82 years old, had been an only child and, having lost his parents, had no known family. He had served with great honour with the Canadian Corps in the First World War and fought in the Battle of Vimy Ridge where so many of his comrades were killed. Returning home, devastated by what he had seen, he withdrew from society and rented a smallholding away from civilisation. Essentially, he became a self-sufficient hermit.

Whilst living in the care home, he made a great impression on the staff. He was old fashioned, had a quiet dignity, was respectful, and always grateful for the care he was given. As the end approached, the staff asked him whom they should contact to make the necessary arrangement, but it appeared there was no-one. There was no next of kin, no family, no friend or neighbour, not even any meaningful acquaintance. It seemed, therefore, that no-one except possibly a funeral director would attend his funeral. Owen spoke of these matters without regret, saying he had lived a solitary life, but one that had suited him. He did, however, express the wish to be buried on the plot that had been his home for the last fifty five years.

Hearing this, Mason was determined that Owen should not be laid to rest without anyone being there to grieve for him. He decided he would make the effort and be present at the burial.

When the day of the funeral arrived, he set off early but unfortunately had a puncture, then got lost trying to find Owen's shack and was unable to find anyone to ask for directions in that wild location.

Eventually, he arrived an hour late. The vicar had already departed, as had the hearse, only the two gravediggers were present, and they were eating their sandwich lunch on a nearby wooden bench. Mason felt bad and apologised to the men for being late, then went to the grave to pay his respects to the hermit who had become his friend.

As he looked down, he saw that the gravediggers had already started to fill the hole, such that the coffin was no longer visible. He didn't quite know what to do but having travelled so far to bid his farewells, he took out his bagpipes and started to play. The gravediggers put down their lunches and gathered around. Mason played heart and soul, as he'd never played before, for this dignified man, who had neither family nor friends.

Having played for some thirty minutes, he finished by playing 'Amazing Grace', a rendering which received a round of applause from the workmen. Mason then packed up his bagpipes and headed back to his pickup. Though his head was hung low, his heart was full, knowing he had done the right thing and made an effort to attend.

As he opened the door of the pickup, he heard one of the workers say, 'I've never seen or heard anything like that before - and I've been putting in septic tanks for over twenty years.'

Thought for the day

'Memorial services are the cocktail parties of the geriatric set.'

Ralph Richardson 1902-1983

An Undeserved Present

I was 27 years old and unemployed. It was a strange new experience for me, and I didn't like it. I was also married with an 18-month-old baby, and another on the way. To make matters worse, after years of living in rented accommodation, my wife and I had recently taken the plunge, put down a deposit on a house, and acquired a mortgage. There were monthly mortgage repayments to be made, and I didn't know where the money was going to come from.

Some might say it was my own fault that I was jobless, as there were plenty of situations available that I could have taken. The problem was that they would all have taken my career backward. Let me explain.

I had set my heart on a career in surgery, despite knowing the voyage ahead would be long and perilous. Even with a fair wind and calm sea, it took a minimum of ten year's training to make the grade of consultant, and that training had to include specific components. I'd just completed a fixed-term contract in a University Hospital, where I had become familiar with the latest medical ideas and research. Now I needed to work in a busy District General Hospital to gain practical 'hands-on' experience; a job in which I would spend a lot of time in the operating theatre, honing my practical surgical skills. Unfortunately, there wasn't one currently available - hence my unemployment. The answer to my financial worries was to obtain a locum job in general practice, until a suitable DGH post became available, and I was pleased when a friend from my student days, offered me an opportunity.

Now I have a confession to make! Young and naive as I was, I'd come to regard general practice as a second-rate medical specialty and general practitioners as second-class doctors. Proper doctors I felt, worked in hospitals! There is actually little excuse for me holding such a view, but by way of partial justification, I should explain that almost all of my medical experience had been spent in a hospital environment; initially as a medical student, then later as a junior doctor. I'd noticed that hospital consultants often spoke of their general practitioner colleagues with a certain disdain. They seemed to regard themselves as superior beings and were prone to comment adversely on the diagnostic skills of GPs and the quality of their referral letters.

I'd witnessed consultants in their clinics throw a GPs letter onto the desk in disgust saying: 'Just look at that; no attempt to make a diagnosis, no background medical history, nothing to say what medication the patient is taking. It's a disgrace. All the GP has written is *Dear Doctor, Re Mrs Betty Jones. Please see and advise!* He's not even had the courtesy to address me by my name!'

As a result, I embarked on my locum GP job eager to impress and keen to demonstrate a higher standard of medicine than they practised. How the mighty are fallen. It only took a few days for me to realise just how different general practice was, and to appreciate the wide range of skills and experience required of a general practitioner. In a hospital there was always the assumption that the patient had a significant illness, and it was our responsibility to diagnose and treat it. In the community, it seemed the opposite was the case; the assumption being that in most cases, there wasn't any significant disease. I saw many patients with coughs and arranged chest x-rays for every one of them; until the senior partner gently pointed out that none of the x-rays I'd arranged showed any abnormality at all.

'If all GPs behaved as you are doing,' he explained, 'we would overwhelm the local x-ray department within a week.'

The same was true for the dozens of blood tests I'd requested, for vague flu-like symptoms.

'But they might have glandular fever or brucellosis,' I argued.

'Yes, they certainly might; but 99% of them won't. Treat their symptoms with paracetamol and a cough bottle,' he advised, 'and ask them to see you in a fortnight if they're not better.'

Of course, he was right, and I quickly came to realise that general practice requires a combination of skill, knowledge, and experience that is quite different to that needed in hospital practice.

One day, I was called to see a lady on a home visit, who had called the surgery complaining she was short of breath. She hadn't been prioritised to be one of my early visits, and I'd organised my round to minimise driving time, so it was late in the day when I reached her.

She was a wiry 75 year-old called Mary Fisher, and the moment I walked through the door, I realised I had a medical emergency on my hands. She was lying on her bed, barely conscious; pale, cold, clammy and acutely breathless. She had experienced some chest pain earlier in the day and was in acute heart failure. It was a situation I had dealt with many times in the past but always in a hospital setting. I quickly realised I had no ECG machine, no oxygen, and no one to turn to should I need assistance.

I did, however, have a medical bag in which I'd put a variety of items that I thought might be useful. These included the standard drugs used at this time to treat heart failure; frusemide, digoxin, and aminophylline. All three were colourless liquids.

With a fair amount of confidence, I opened the three glass vials and placed them on the small bedside table. Then I delved into my back for needles and syringes. There were plenty of needles - but only one syringe. No matter, I thought, I'll draw up the aminophylline and then mix in the digoxin and frusemide. After all, I reasoned, it's all going to be injected intravenously. But disaster struck. When I added the digoxin and frusemide to the clear solution of aminophylline, it turned into a white mixture, which then congealed in the syringe to the consistency of thick yoghurt. I placed the needle in Mrs Fisher's vein but no matter how hard I pushed on the plunger, the mixture was too thick to inject through the needle.

By this time, the patient was deteriorating rapidly, her husband was getting increasingly concerned, and I was getting more red-faced and embarrassed as every minute passed. I was fearful that at any moment, I should have a death on my hands.

'Dial 999 for an ambulance' I instructed her husband, hoping the rising panic I felt did not show in my voice, 'and stress to them it's very urgent.'

I sat with the patient until the paramedics came. They gave her oxygen, popped her onto a stretcher, and whisked her off to hospital.

Later that evening, now back at home, I had time to reflect on what had happened. To err is to be human. No one goes through their career, whatever their calling, without making mistakes. Anyone who claims that they have is a liar. What is important is to learn from mistakes, and to avoid repeating them. I vowed to take greater care in future when preparing my medical bag. Some mistakes have severe consequences but in this instance. I'd been fortunate. What had happened had shaken me up, embarrassed me, but luckily the patient had come to no harm.

A greater embarrassment occurred a fortnight later when I visited

Mrs Fisher after she had been discharged from hospital, having survived her myocardial infarction. Her husband forced a bottle of whisky on me, whilst Mrs Fisher embraced me in a bearlike hug, kissed me on both cheeks and, with tears in her eyes, thanked me for saving her life!

Thought for the day

Pride cometh before a fall
Book of Proverbs

Charles D. Forbes Comes of Age

Orthopaedic surgeons are often caricatured as carefree, larger than life, confident characters, built like international rugby players, who work on their patients with hammers, saws, and chisels, with all the finesse of a Japanese sumo wrestler. Charles D. Forbes however, was most definitely not of that ilk. Slightly built, with a gentle, unassuming manner, he was the kindest, gentlest man you could care to meet. Invariably polite, never one to argue, he simply got on with his job in a calm, quiet and efficient manner.

It was these characteristics, however, laudable as they were, that were the cause of his greatest unhappiness, for everyone took advantage of his forgiving nature and his inability to say 'no'. Whenever there were extra patients to be seen in the hospital's outpatient clinic, the clerical staff invariably added them to his list. This frequently resulted in him remaining at work, long after his colleagues had gone off duty. At home, his wife and daughters assumed that he would always play second fiddle, acting as chauffeur, gardener and scullery maid, whilst they pursued their various interests and hobbies – and spent the money that he earned! Even when trying to enjoy his only form of relaxation, a game of golf, he was plagued by fellow club members, who expected him to give his medical opinion of their various aches and pains, both on the course and in the clubhouse.

Being a patient and forgiving man, he tolerated this abuse without complaint for many years, but all the while, anger, and resentment were building up inside him, like a volcano ready to erupt. Eventually, the pressure became unbearable; he decided that enough was enough. He had reached breaking point. He realised that if he didn't sort his life out, he would be downtrodden for the rest of his days.

Not a man to act in anger, in haste, or without forethought, he deliberated for many weeks before deciding on his plan of campaign. His actions had to be reasonable, must certainly not cause anyone any distress or hardship, he definitely wouldn't want that, but equally, they should leave people in no doubt that the days of treating him as a doormat were over. Then, having formulated his plan, he had to decide when it would be implemented. He settled on his birthday, which happened to be following Friday.

As the big day approached, any fears that he would get cold feet at the last minute melted away, as he reflected on all the years he had put others before himself. He became ever more certain he was justified in taking action and was doing the right thing.

On Friday morning, nervous but determined, he went to work as usual. He completed his morning theatre session, had lunch with colleagues then went to the outpatient clinic. Before seeing his first patient, he called at the reception desk.

'I'm afraid I have to be off on the dot of five today,' he said, 'so please don't add any extra patients to my list.'

'But I've already added a couple,' came the reply from the receptionist, fully expecting Mr Forbes to agree to see them. 'One is a woman who should have come yesterday but forgot the appointment; the other is a patient that Mr Brown didn't have time to see this morning.'

'I'm afraid that you'll have to make alternative arrangements,' Mr Forbes replied.

'But what shall I do with these two patients? They're expecting to see you.'

'I'm sorry,' the consultant said, wondering why he kept apologising when he had nothing to apologise for, 'but that's something for you to decide. My list is already full, and regrettably today, I'm not available after five.'

He could feel his heart beating hard in his chest but he kept his voice quiet and controlled. 'If you'd asked me, I would have told you that I wasn't able to see any extra patients today. In future, that is what I'd like you to do.'

Mr Forbes waited for a minute or two in his consulting room allowing his pulse to settle, before calling for his first patient. He felt pleased; part one of his plan had gone well. He knew, though, that part two, dealing with his wife and family might be more difficult.

Sally was surprised when her husband arrived home a good hour earlier than usual.

'The clinic was a little quieter than usual,' he explained. 'If dinner is at the usual time, I think I'll potter in the garden; it's been a bit neglected recently.'

'No, don't do that,' his wife replied. 'Peel the potatoes and carrots for me; I just need to get to the end of this book, then you'll be able to drop it off at the library for me in the morning.'

But she found herself talking to an empty room; Charles was already on his way to the potting shed.

An hour later, the evening meal was taken in an uneasy silence but nothing untoward was said about the vegetables, and Charles noticed with satisfaction that the next time Sally wanted a job doing it was a case of, 'If you're free, would you mind....'

His major success though came the next day at the golf club. The club secretary, Sam Cartwright, sidled up to him in the bar, where Charles was having a quiet drink with friends after a pleasant morning's game. Sam, who was a somewhat officious club employee, whose overzealous application of club rules had upset a number of club members, started to quiz him about his painful knee.

'Do you want me to have a look at it for you?' Charles asked.

Sam jumped at the offer.

'Right, come with me.'

Charles led Sam to the Gents locker room where other club members were changing into and out of their golf gear. There he took a detailed history, including asking some personal questions about the secretary's smoking and drinking habits. Then he instructed Sam to strip to his underpants.

Sam was taken by surprise; he hadn't expected to undress to be examined.

'What... here, is that really necessary?' Sam protested, suddenly remembering he hadn't changed his underpants for a couple of days, and realising that this could be very embarrassing.

'Yes, it is necessary,' Mr Forbes replied, 'pain felt in the knee may be due to a knee problem, but it can also be a referred pain from a condition in the lumbar region or hip. You asked me for my opinion, so yes, I do need to examine you.'

By this time, quite a number of club members had gathered, and Sam began to feel a little awkward. Perhaps it hadn't been such a good idea to ask for a free medical opinion.

'Look, I didn't really expect....' he began.

'It's really no trouble at all, and I'm sure you want me to do the job properly.'

Wearing only a pair of rather grey boxers, Charles had the secretary walking the length of the locker room; 'I need to see if you have a limp', he explained.

Sam was then required to lie on his back on one of the benches whilst Charles checked for pain during movements of his hip and knee joints. As the clinical examination progressed, Sam's embarrassment increased, as did the number of spectators, quite a number of them pleased to witness Sam's discomfiture.

'Look, you mustn't go to all this trouble; let's call it a....' he spluttered.

'It's really no trouble, and we're nearly through now,' Charles replied, before commencing on a full assessment of the secretary's back which involved touching his toes, arching and rotating his spine and finally a full neurological examination of his lower limbs, including such minutia as having Sam say whether his toes were being moved upwards or downwards with his eyes blindfolded. The assembled crowd loved it and even started to suggest additional humiliations that might be heaped upon the unfortunate man.

'I've got a needle; you could use it to see if he can feel pain.'

'What about a rectal examination. I've heard that piles can sometimes cause pain in the knee.'

Finally, his examination complete, Charles gave Sam his verdict. 'It's no more than a little bit of arthritis. Only what can be expected for a man of your age who is overweight. It's really nothing to worry about.'

Afterward, it was a rather subdued club secretary who returned to the bar. 'Look, I really ought to buy you a drink,' he said, to thank you for your trouble.

'That's very kind,' Charles replied, 'a double whisky would go down a treat, and I'll pop the bill in the post for you!'

And he did. A bill for £150 for the consultation arrived for the club secretary within the week, and that, together with the frequent retelling of the story on the golf club grapevine, ensured that Charles was never asked for free medical advice again.

A Visit to London

Joe was not relishing the prospect of the trip to London; England's capital was not his favourite city. It was not that he disliked the people who lived there; it was simply that he associated London with stress and anxiety, interviews and examinations, cheap hotels and plastic food. His aversion resulted from an unsuccessful application, made many years previously, for a place at the medical school of one of London's oldest and most prestigious teaching hospitals.

At the time, as a naive 'A' level student, he was making his first trip to the city. His train had arrived at Euston station an hour and a half late, thanks to a signalling failure at Crewe. Then, there had been a further delay on the Northern Line of the Underground. In an attempt to make up time, he had run the last half mile to the medical school, through wind and rain, and arrived hot, breathless, wet and agitated. He found the Dean's Office, where the interviews were to be held, and introduced himself to the Dean's secretary.

'You're late,' she said, then showed him to a small room where half a dozen other candidates were sitting-waiting to be interviewed. All were smartly dressed, some in school uniform, others in dark suits; the girls wore black skirts and neat blouses.

Before he had time to compose himself, his name was called, and he was ushered into an oak-panelled committee room. He hadn't even had the chance to take off his wet coat. Across a large oak desk, he came face to face with two crusty-looking, elderly gentlemen, whose facial expressions were as severe as those of the unsmiling figures depicted in the gold-framed portraits on the wall behind them. Presumably, these were past consultants of the hospital, now long dead, and no longer able to terrorise aspiring young doctors, such as Joe.

The older of the two gentlemen regarded Joe over the rim of his half-moon glasses. His thin white hair, lined face, hollow cheeks, and gaunt appearance suggested that it might not be long before he too was immortalised in a framed portrait. He spoke in a clipped, high-pitched, wavering voice.

'Now what have we got here?' The use of the word *'what'*

instead of 'who', together with the querulous tone of his voice, suggested this was less of a question addressed to Joe, more a comment to his colleague.

He adjusted his glasses then peered at the papers in front of him.

'So, you're Barnes, are you, David Barnes?'

'No, Sir, my name is Beddows, Sir.'

'Meadows did you say?' he responded, a hand cupped to his ear.

'No, Sir, Beddows, Joseph Beddows,' Joe replied, speaking a little louder and as clearly as he could.

'Did you say Beddows? You really shouldn't mumble my boy. You must learn to speak more distinctly.'

'Yes, sir, Beddows.'

The old man looked down again and made an amendment to the notes in front of him.

'I see. So you're young Beddows, are you? I take it you're Rupert Beddows' grandson from Winchester. How is your grandfather keeping these days? Does he still do a spot of fishing?'

He turned to his colleague. 'Rupert and I were pals at college in the old days. We played a lot of rugger together. Did you know we were both in the team that won the London Hospital Shield? He was centre, I played on the wing. Those were good days.'

'No, sir, I'm Joseph Beddows from Accrington.'

The elderly gent frowned and consulted his notes again.

'We weren't expecting a Beddows; you should be Barnes, David Barnes. What are you doing here?'

A doubt entered Joe's mind. He had arrived at the last minute in a fluster. Was it possible that he was in the wrong place?

'I've applied for a place at the medical school, Sir. Your secretary took my name and escorted me in here.'

The interviewer, who had addressed him but failed to introduce himself, conferred with his equally anonymous colleague. He had unfashionably long, grey hair that hung down in untidy strands over his collar. He wore a velvet jacket and a red and white spotted bow tie. Joe marked him down as a retired psychiatrist. He was possibly a couple of years younger than his partner though still looked to be nearer eighty than seventy. Then the older man spoke again.

'We were expecting to see Barnes next. His father is the Professor of Orthopaedics here, you know,' he added as an aside. 'I really don't understand what can have happened. Applicants are supposed to come in here in alphabetical order, but I do see there is a 'Beddows' on our list.'

There was further conferring and more shuffling of papers. Joe felt a growing irritation. It seemed obvious to him that Barnes had either cancelled or been delayed, and that Beddows was the next name on their list.

'So you're Beddows, are you, from Accrington did you say?'

Joe confirmed, again, that was indeed the case.

'That's in Lancashire, isn't it, somewhere north of Manchester?'

From the grimace on his face, and the sideways glance at his colleague, Joe gained the impression that, in his mind, Manchester was the limit of the known world, beyond which civilisation ceased to exist.

Joe nodded.

'I don't think we've had anyone from Accrington before,' his interviewer remarked to no one in particular. 'And you aspire to study medicine here?' he questioned, managing to instil a tone of incredulity into his voice.

He regarded Joe's windswept hair. Then his eyes swept over his wet raincoat, which was dripping water to form a small puddle on the polished parquet floor. He sniffed as he noted Joe's trousers, damp from the knee down and his best black school shoes, the ones he had cleaned, brushed and polished so assiduously before leaving home but which were now mud-splattered and scuffed.

He sniffed again. 'Well, Beddows,' he said, disapproval evident in his voice, 'if you wish to be considered for a career in medicine, I must advise you that medicine is a highly respectable profession. We expect a certain minimum standard of dress and behaviour. Our patients expect us to be appropriately attired at all times. What do you imagine a solicitor or bank manager would think if they came to consult you for a medical opinion and found you looking so....' he paused, searching for the right word, '....dishevelled? The purpose of these interviews is to ensure that we only admit the right sort of chap. You do understand that, I suppose?'

'Yes, Sir,' Joe replied. 'I do apologise for my appearance. Unfortunately, my train was delayed. It has been quite a rush to get here, and it is raining rather heavily outside.'

'Our patients also expect us to make contingency plans to ensure that we always fulfil our appointments. You should have travelled down last night, shouldn't you?'

'Yes, Sir,' Joe replied. He could have countered this criticism on the grounds of expense but decided that any further attempt to justify himself would be counter-productive.

With that, his assessor sniffed yet again, jotted some notes on the pad in front of him, then turned to his colleague.

'I don't think I have any more questions for this fellow, Charles. Is there anything that you wish to ask?'

The younger of the two geriatrics eyed Joe quizzically, as a cat might eye a mouse, wondering whether to kill it straight away or to have some fun before doing so. He decided on the latter course.

'Tell me, Beddows, what's life like in Accrington?'

Joe was at a loss to know what to say. He had never been in such a situation before and had received no guidance on interview technique, either from his parents or at school. When trying to predict the questions that he might face, he had anticipated there might be a reference to his academic record, his selection as head boy, his interests, sporting activities, and hobbies. He thought perhaps they might ask his reasons for wishing to study medicine, but not about life in Accrington.

'Well, Sir,' he managed to reply after a longish pause, 'It suits me well enough. I'm happy there. But it's the only town in which I've lived; I really have nothing with which to compare it.'

'Happy in Accrington, eh? Surely not.' The interviewer looked across at his colleague, smiled sadly then turned back to Joe.

'Perhaps that shows a certain lack of ambition,' he commented. 'Have you given any thought of studying perhaps in Manchester, Leeds or Liverpool, for example?'

'I have ambitions to study medicine in London, Sir,' Joe replied stiffly, angered by the tone of the question.

'Ah, yes, but should those ambitions not be realised, would Manchester or Liverpool suffice?'

It was obvious he was being told that his application was unsuccessful. They had evidently taken one look at him, heard his North Country accent and decided he was not suitable for their precious teaching hospital. The interview continued for a further two or three minutes during which time, they ascertained that there was no opera, ballet or concert hall in Accrington before they politely showed him the door. Why, Joe wondered, had they had bothered to drag him all the way down to London for an interview if they were going to dismiss him so abruptly? Was it perhaps because he happened to have the same surname as one of his interviewer's old

Winchester college friend?

The gathering dusk, a developing fog, and the continuing rain added to Joe's gloom as he left the hospital and turned towards the tube station. As he did so, a huge road sign confronted him. It showed a large black arrow pointing along the road on which he was walking. In the most enormous letters was written 'THE NORTH'. That just about sums it up, he thought. Go back where you belong, young man, London is not for you.

The Music Festival

I really don't know how I came to fall, but I did. Our two boys were away at their annual summer Scout camp, so my wife and I had decided, at short notice, to slip away for a short weekend break. We'd both been working hard and felt we deserved it. We drove to the delightful village of Edale in Derbyshire and booked into Bed and Breakfast accommodation; lodgings we'd enjoyed on a previous visit. On the Saturday, a day of sunshine and showers, we did little more than potter around the village and treat ourselves to some pub grub in the evening.

The weather forecast for the Sunday was for fine, sunny weather, so we set off to climb Kinder Scout. We followed the well-trodden path up Jacob's Ladder and reached the top without difficulty. There we ate our sandwiches but didn't linger, for the mountain top really isn't at all attractive. There isn't a summit as such; the top is flat, at least a mile across and essentially is an expanse of wet, peaty marshland, crisscrossed by gullies, deep enough to hide a full-grown man.

It was on the way down that I came a cropper. To this day, I don't know how it happened; perhaps I simply wasn't looking where I was going, but one minute I was strolling along without a care in the world, the next I was flying, head-over-heels, onto the stony path. I escaped with a bruise on my forehead, wounded pride and broken glasses; they had snapped across the bridge. I dusted myself off and assured my wife that I hadn't come to any serious harm. Then I patched up my glasses with some adhesive plaster from my first aid kit and resolved to be more careful in the future. We continued on our way and completed the walk without further incident.

The day after we returned home, I again packed my bags, and my Wellington boots, this time for a trip to Somerset. For the last three years, I've acted as a medical officer for a well-known music festival. In truth, it doesn't pay well, but it's always an interesting experience and makes a refreshing change from my normal life as a country General Practitioner.

I form part of a small team of doctors, nurses, and paramedics from both the county ambulance service and the St John's

Ambulance Brigade. Our brief is to provide immediate resuscitation and triage should an emergency arise in the crowd, who incidentally, are monitored on closed-circuit television rather more closely than they may imagine. We are supported by a 'snatch squad'. They are able to dive into the mass of partygoers, many of whom are fuelled with alcohol and drugs, hoist out anyone who collapses and bring them post-haste to our resuscitation tent, which is situated behind the main stage. It wasn't long before I received a message in my radio earplug, to say they were bringing in an unconscious collapsed male in his late-20s.

He arrived two minutes later. We had no couches at the forward posts, so the stretcher was laid on the floor, and I knelt down to assess him with a primary and secondary survey. I had to adjust my glasses which were sitting rather cock-eyed on my nose.

Most of the festival-goers who needed treatment had problems due to a combination of alcohol, opiates, diazepam derivatives, amphetamines, and dehydration. This man was moderately deep with a Glasgow Coma Score of 5-6. He was hypoventilating and his oxygen saturation level was low. I set up an intravenous line, administered fluids, and gave him some initial Naloxone. Anxiously, I knelt over him to judge his response. I needed to decide whether he could stay on-site, or if he required transfer to the local hospital for more intensive treatment. A paramedic and several others in the tent watched, equally concerned.

Slowly, he started to stir, then gradually opened his eyes. He gazed up, looking at me intently. He then started to speak in long, drawn-out syllables, accentuating his words with vague uncoordinated movements of his arms.

'Yooooouuuuu' he said very slowly, 'neeeeeeed....' he paused, 'tooo goooh too....' a longer pause, his arms still waving vaguely in the air... SpecSavers.'

This rather unexpected comment caused great hilarity within the ranks. Our patient then passed out again, and we continued with his resuscitation until success was finally achieved.

I took my glasses for repair the next day.

(Based on a story by Dr Ian Gibson)

Thought for the day

Cocaine habit forming? Of course not. I ought to know. I've been using it for years.   Tallulah Bankhead 1903 - 1968

A Good Night Out

It was the occasion of the Unit's Christmas night out; the night on which the staff who had worked so hard throughout the year on the wards and in the theatres, could let their hair down and enjoy themselves. Everyone who had contributed to the success of the unit was invited; nurses, doctors, physiotherapists, porters, cleaners, and secretaries. It was a much anticipated event and a great way of breaking down social barriers amongst the staff. Many of the other units held their annual party in the hospital, but the head of the orthopaedic unit knew from previous experience, that this was unwise. If the staff were to relax, have a drink, and enjoy themselves, it was better that this should happen away from the watchful eyes of the patients and visitors.

The senior consultant in charge of the unit was Mr Daffyd Llewellyn Jones, a fierce and domineering Welshman who, though short in stature, walked the wards with his head held high, running his unit with a rod of iron. He was sometimes referred to, though not in his presence, as D L J. Just as frequently though, he was simply called God. There was only one way of managing any given bony injury, and that was His way. His rules for the treatment of fractures were issued to all members of staff in the form of a small black book, which inevitably was known as The Bible. Follow the instructions in The Bible, and you escaped trouble, even if the patient's convalescence was complicated by some terrible disaster. Break the rules, and you were in dire straits, even if the patient made a full recovery in a fraction of the expected time.

D L J also worked at the Fairfield Hospital, a smaller hospital in a neighbouring town, and his favourite phrase when reprimanding staff at the main hospital was *'You're the worst ...... I've ever known. The ...... at the Fairfield are so much better than you.'* The blanks could be filled with the word 'nurse', 'doctor', or 'porter' depending on the circumstance. The previous year's annual 'get together' had been a combined affair, and the staff from the two hospitals had come together for the first time. Inevitably, the occasion was an opportunity for reminiscing and swopping stories. When someone mentioned they got irritated by constantly being told how superb the Fairfield staff were, all the Fairfield staff fell about laughing.

'He's obviously playing us off against each other,' they said. 'He tells us we're the worst he's ever known, and how you lot are so much better than we are!'

Although these characteristics made him a hard taskmaster, he was always fiercely loyal to the members of his team. He worked them hard, taught them well, and if they measured up to his high standards, he supported them regardless of the situation. He might well berate them when they were working for him, but he would defend them to the death, should they be criticised by outsiders.

The staff party was held in a night club in the city centre. Ken Robson, the orthopaedic registrar, supported by one of the housemen, was left in charge in the hospital. D L J, a bachelor who was teetotal thanks to his strict Welsh Methodist upbringing, would be available at home should any problem arise that Ken was unable to manage.

The party was a great success, with a great deal of singing and dancing, laughter and drinking and was enjoyed by all. It didn't break up until one in the morning. Meanwhile, back at the hospital, no serious problems arose on the wards, and the casualty department was also quiet. There was, therefore, no need for Ken to disturb his boss at home. However, shortly after one-thirty, he was called to casualty to attend the victims of a road traffic accident. To his dismay, he found that one of the injured drivers was Geoff Norton, the Senior Registrar on the Unit, who was second in command to D L J himself. Fortunately, no one was seriously hurt and Ken was able to patch them up without too much trouble. Regrettably though, Geoff was, in the parlance of the time, 'under the influence'.

Whilst he was being treated in casualty, the police arrived wishing to speak to the drivers of the cars involved. Sensing trouble, Ken phoned D L J.

'Take Norton immediately to the office at the back of the operating theatre' was the instruction, 'I'm on my way.'

D L J lived twenty minutes away but arrived in fifteen.

'Where's Norton?' he demanded, the minute he arrived. 'Did you manage to get him into the theatre?'

'Yes, Sir, I did,' Ken replied.

'Right Robson, come with me.'

Quickly, they made their way to the theatre, entering via the back door.

Ten minutes later, the police found their way to the orthopaedic unit and asked to speak with the senior doctor in charge. They were told he was in the operating theatre. D L J met them at the theatre door, now wearing his green theatre vest and pants.

'I am the Professor of Orthopaedics,' he announced, even though he wasn't. 'I am just about to deal with my injured colleague and I'm afraid he will not be able to talk with anyone until the morning.'

Ken noted that the boss was careful to say 'deal with' rather than 'operate upon'!

D L J then did indeed proceed to 'deal with' Norton in no uncertain fashion in the office.

Ken returned to the doctor's mess to relay the story to his friends, a story that would be told and retold in the hospital for many years to come. The police left empty-handed!

(Based on a story by Mr Ken Tuson)

<u>Thought for the day</u>

But I'm not so think as you drunk I am.

J. C. Squire 1884 - 1958

Getting Even

A small extension was being built at the rear of the Park Lane Surgery. Over the years, the number of patients on the General Practitioners list had increased, an additional partner had been appointed, and she needed a consulting room. The extension would also increase the waiting area for patients, and provide an office for the practice manager. The work was being undertaken by a small local firm called Simpson and Webb, chosen because Bob Simpson was a great friend of Tony Grainger, the son of the senior partner. Bob, desperate to pay off the overdraft extended to him from the bank when he had set up his small building company a couple of years before, had promised to do as much of the work as possible, and certainly the bulk of the noisy disruptive work, at weekends to minimise any disturbance to the doctors.

All was going well until the third week in July. The site had been cleared, the foundations dug, and the brickwork completed to the level of the windows. Then the calamity occurred. It happened one day while Bob and his partner, Jim Webb, were busy bricklaying at the back of the surgery. A sneak thief took the opportunity to steal valuable equipment from Bob's white van, which had been parked at the front. Bob was furious; he lost a generator, a small compressor, an angle grinder and a number of electric power tools. He reckoned it would cost the best part of £2000 to replace what had been stolen, money he simply did not have. To make matters worse, he was not insured; that had been a calculated risk, taken to reduce his overheads. He cursed his stupidity for leaving his van unlocked and unattended.

Inevitably, he reported his loss to the police who logged the incident, made sympathetic noises, said they would make some enquiries, but suggested that the chances of the equipment being recovered were slim. They did, however, suggest that Bob keep an eye out for his tools, both at local car boot sales and on eBay.

***

Fast forward three weeks, during which time Bob fumed at his misfortune, but gradually became resigned to his loss. Not having the means to replace the stolen items with new, he was making do

184

with equipment purchased second-hand or borrowed from friends, but life wasn't easy. Every job seemed to take longer than before and, as always in the building trade, time costs money. He was busy fixing the double-glazed window units into place when his mobile phone rang.

'Hello,' said a rough male voice that he didn't recognise. 'Is that Bob Simpson, builder and property repairer?'

'Yes, it is,' said Bob, his hopes rising; perhaps this was someone who might offer him a contract.

'What can I do to help you?'

'Are you the fella' that had some stuff nicked from your van recently?'

'Yes, I am,' Bob answered eagerly. 'Are you the police? Have you found the equipment that was stolen?'

'Yes, I've got your tools and stuff mate; it's safe and sound' the voice laughed, 'but I....

'Why that's wonderful,' Bob interrupted, greatly relieved. Now he would be able to get back to normal.

The laugh on the phone continued, '....but I'm not the police – far from it.'

'Well, who are you then?'

'I'm the fella' what nicked it.'

'You what....?'

'I told you, I'm the fella' what nicked it.'

'You bastard.'

'Hey – no hard feelings, mate. But if you leave your gear on show at the side of the road, you really shouldn't be surprised if it disappears.'

'Those tools are my property, you bastard. I want them back.'

Quickly he glanced at the phone's screen. '*Number withheld',* he read and cursed again.

'Well, you can have your tools back. They're not much use to me, they're very poor quality. The truth is, if I'd known they were such rubbish, I'd never have bothered nicking them in the first place! I've tried to sell them in the pub, on the net, car boot sales, all over the place - but nobody wants them. I can't get rid of them anywhere. It's bloody annoying. When I think of all the time I've wasted trying to get a bob or two for them, I wish now I'd never gone to the bother of nicking them.'

'Those tools are bloody good tools. The generator alone cost me over a grand – you damn well bring them back.'

'I'll not be giving them back after all the effort I've spent trying to offload them, but if you were to make me an offer for them, we might be talking.'

'What! You mean me buy my own tools back from you, when you've stolen them from me in the first place - you've got a bloody nerve!'

'You were the one who said they were valuable. Now you be sensible, you make me an offer. If it's a fair offer, I'll not refuse it.'

'Get lost.'

'Suppose you give me, let's say ....three hundred....quid....' but then the words on the other end of the line became great guffaws of uncontrollable laughter. When it subsided, the voice returned, now softer and more cultured.

'Bob, hey Bob, just calm down and listen for a moment, will you? Do you know a guy called Tony Grainger, son of the doctor on Park Lane? Isn't he your best friend?'

'Yes, I know Bob, what the hell's that to you.'

'Well, Bob, my name's Tommy West, I'm the DJ on the afternoon slot on Radio Liverpool. Your pal, Tony, contacted us a day or two ago and suggested that we gave you a ring for our '*get your own back*' spot. Didn't you embarrass him on his stag night, arranging a little tattoo on his backside, when he'd had one drink too many?"

'So, this is all a bloody wind-up. I'll kill that bastard when I can get hold of him.'

'Now, now, Bob, I think we've had enough 'effing and blinding' for one afternoon, don't you. The bleep machine we use to blank out 'f words' is already going to be working overtime before we can get this transcript ready for broadcasting. But thanks for being such a good sport.'

'You're not going to broadcast this are you?'

'Oh, yes, we are. It's the best wind up we've had in years – great entertainment for our listeners. We shall just need a good song to go with it; perhaps that song by the great Country and Western singer, Johnny Cash; 'You're my best friend.'

After all these years of fishing, the fish are having their revenge.

> Queen Elizabeth, the Queen Mother after an operation to remove a fishbone stuck in her throat 1900 – 2002

Lunch with a Lovely Lady

I wasn't best pleased when called to the phone. I don't like being disturbed when I'm working, particularly when I'm conducting a delicate examination to decide whether a lady's piles require surgery.

'An outside call for you, Dr Trotter,' said the telephonist. 'It sounds like a young lady, but she wouldn't give me her name; she said it was personal.'

'Hello there, this is Suzie,' the voice said when the call was connected. It was a cheerful young voice, but not one I recognised; nor indeed did I know anyone called Suzie!

I must have paused, for she continued, 'Don't you remember? We met in the clinic yesterday when I brought Julie to see you. You operated on her as an emergency about a month ago.'

Suddenly, I did remember. Julie was the 10-year-old daughter of a well-to-do family. Theirs was a fancy address in a local village that had become fashionable with over-paid footballers and stockbrokers. Her father was a banker or some such in the city. Julie had been admitted as an emergency about a month before with abdominal pain. The diagnosis of appendicitis had been easy enough to make; the difficulty had been her father, who insisted the operation be performed by a consultant surgeon in a private hospital. However, try as he might, at 1 am on a Sunday morning, he hadn't been able to find a consultant available to do it.

By this stage in my career, I had performed dozens of appendix operations. Julie was slim and otherwise healthy, and I felt sufficiently competent to crack on, to remove the offending organ, and then get to my bed. However, Julie's Dad expressed concern about my age and what he considered to be my relative inexperience. Quite a delay ensued before I felt obliged to issue an ultimatum; either Julie remains in pain, getting more toxic by the minute as you prevaricate, or I take her to theatre and do what needs to be done.

With considerable reluctance and only after a detailed discussion of the procedure and the associated surgical and anaesthetic risks, did he agree to sign the consent form. Fortunately, his fears about my surgical ability proved to be unfounded, the operation was completed without incident, and Julie's recovery was unremarkable.

She was now fit and well.

Perhaps unsurprisingly, I remembered Suzie as well; she was Julie's elder sister. Slim and attractive, probably 19 or 20 years of age, she had sparkling eyes and a ready smile. She had turned the heads of many of the male staff when visiting Julie in hospital, not least because of her long legs and miniskirts.

I was surprised that she had rung me and wondered what she wanted. Were there some further questions about Julie she wished to discuss or had they perhaps inadvertently left something behind in the clinic? But her next remark astonished me.

'David, I may call you David, mayn't I? I hope this isn't an inconvenient time to call, but I thought it would be nice if we were to go out for a meal together sometime.'

At the time, I considered myself to be an overworked, over-tired, rather introverted, dull bachelor, not one who found it easy to ask a girl for a date. To have this gorgeous young lady ring me out of the blue and suggest a rendezvous, left me temporarily speechless.

'Well, yes, that would be very pleasant,' I eventually managed to stutter.

Thanks to my hospital duty roster, we had some difficulty fixing the date but finally settled on lunch, one day during the following week. Suzie said she would look forward to it and would arrange a reservation at her favourite restaurant. I returned to my duties in the clinic in a somewhat distracted state, wondering what the future had in store for me.

When we met for our date, Suzie looked stunning. Smiling, she gave me a peck on the cheek, and I felt proud to be the man at her side as we strolled into the restaurant.

Suzie was clearly a regular; the staff greeted her by name and showed us to a reserved table for two in a quiet corner. The white linen table cloth was freshly laundered, and the matching serviettes had been delicately folded into the shape of a fan. There was enough cut glass and silver cutlery at each place setting for a five-course banquet. I began to have concerns; it looked frightfully expensive and, because it was the end of the month, my funds were low. These were the days when it was customary for the gentleman to pay for the lady.

When asked to order pre-dinner drinks, she simply said, 'My usual, please,' and a glass of white wine appeared. I ordered a beer, then immediately wondered if it would have been more appropriate to have ordered wine – not that I should have known which wine to select.

I felt ill at ease and out of my comfort zone in these expensive surroundings, but Suzie seemed relaxed and chatted cheerfully about nothing in particular. When the menu arrived, my fears increased. Whenever I ate out, and I didn't dine out often, I never paid as much for the main course as they were asking here for a starter. I chose the tomato soup, the cheapest item on the menu but to my horror, Suzie selected the crab salad, from the 'specials board' without knowing the cost.

Worried though I was about my finances, I had to admit that Suzie made a delightful companion. She was bright, cheerful, and witty, was obviously widely travelled, and if she noticed my limited knowledge of music and the arts, she was too polite to comment.

'I don't normally eat a large lunch,' she said, as she ordered Beef Wellington, asparagus and dauphinoise potatoes for her main course. I chose a beef burger and wasn't surprised when it came with a fancy salad and a tasty mayonnaise sauce, which I presumed enabled them to justify the exorbitant price they were charging!

I realised with a sense of foreboding that I didn't have enough cash on me to cover the bill. I was even fearful the overdraft limit on my credit card wouldn't cover the damage that was being inflicted on my finances.

As we ate, Suzie showed a keen interest in my life as a trainee surgeon. What did it actually feel like to perform an operation, she wanted to know; how did I cope with the responsibility, and how long would it be before I became a consultant? Speaking of things that were of interest and importance to me, I was able to relax. In turn, she told me about her hobbies; riding, walking, and sailing. There we had a common interest, as I was a competent dinghy sailor and we had a lively discussion about the relative merits of the Enterprise, Wayfarer and GP 14. Suddenly, I found that I was at ease and enjoying myself; Suzie was not only extremely pretty but wonderful company.

As we tucked into our desserts; Strawberries Arnaud for her, plain ice for me, I began to think about how wonderful it would be if our friendship could flourish. I determined that at the end of the meal, I would overcome my natural reserve and suggest another meeting. It would have to be something that wouldn't break the bank, of course, perhaps a walk in the country followed by a meal in a pub. And if that were a success, maybe we could....

My dreams, though, were interrupted as the waiter came to clear away the dessert dishes. We ordered coffee and rounded off our meal with mints and petit fours. Now was the time to suggest that second date.

'Look,' I began, 'I've really enjoyed our lunch together, perhaps we....'

But at that moment, the Maitre D' arrived and placed the bill on the table beside me. I reached for it with a sinking heart but, as quick as a flash, Suzie took it from me. For a second, our hands touched, and butterflies fluttered in my chest.

'I'll take that,' she said.

'No, I should pick up the tab,' I said, desperately hoping that she wouldn't take me up the offer, 'It really has been a very pleasant lunch.'

She looked me in the eye and gave me her sweetest smile. 'No, Mummy's paying for this. Whenever she met you, when you were caring for Julie, she thought you looked half-starved and completely exhausted. She wanted to thank you for what you did for her. My parents were terribly worried when they couldn't find a consultant to perform Julie's operation; they realised afterward they were wrong to suggest you weren't competent to do it. Mummy said I was to take you out, make a fuss of you and give you a hearty meal!'

Susie paid the bill, left the staff a generous tip, then collected her coat, gave me a second peck on the cheek, and left.

With my ego completely deflated, I walked slowly back to the hospital – and I never saw her again.

Thought for the day

Blessed is the man who expects nothing, for he shall never be disappointed.

Alexander Pope 1688 – 1744

St George's Street

It had been a long day; the morning's clinic had overrun, an emergency had been added to the afternoon's operating list, and dusk was falling when I went back to the office to collect my coat. My secretary had already gone home, but she had pinned a message to the lapel of my jacket.

'Sorry, but Dr Bennett rang asking if you would do a D V.
Mrs Edith Smith, aged 80
6 St George's Rd
Obvious breast cancer but probably too frail for surgery.'

The Domiciliary Visiting service is an admirable arrangement that allows General Practitioners to request a specialist to visit a patient at their home. In the early days, I always met the GP in the patient's home, and we undertook the consultation together. Later, due to time constraints, I usually visited on my own. Either way, it was an excellent way of establishing good working relationships with colleagues in General Practice. An additional benefit was that it helped to reduce the number of unnecessary hospital admissions.

I looked through the window at the dark November evening. It was cold and had just started to rain. Finding the address and seeing the patient would delay me by at least an hour. I was tempted to defer the visit; the thought of switching off, and relaxing over a hot meal and a glass of wine in the warmth and comfort of my own home was appealing. However, a quick look at my diary confirmed that the following day already looked busy. I groaned, muttered a vague obscenity, then reluctantly set off to visit Mrs Smith on my way home.

Mrs Smith's home proved to be a 'two-up, two-down' terraced house, with the front door opening straight on to the street. The house was in complete darkness. I knocked but got no response. I knocked again, louder this time, but still, there was no response. The rain was heavier now. I turned up my collar and hammered even harder.

I was just turning to leave, frustrated and angry that I'd made a wasted journey when a figure approached pushing a pram.

'Are you the doctor?' she asked.

I confirmed that I was.

'The key's just inside the box,' she said. 'Just let yourself in.'

I had forgotten that frail elderly folk often hung their front door key on a string just inside the letterbox, so that family, neighbours, or carers were able to gain entrance.

I slipped my hand through the letterbox, hoping there wasn't an aggressive dog loose in the house, located the string with the key attached, and let myself in. The door opened directly into the front room, which in darkness, as indeed was the back room. However, some light was filtering down the stairwell between the two downstairs rooms. Mounting the stairs, I entered a small bedroom. Most of the space was occupied by a large double bed which was hard up against the far wall, and, lying in the bed, was a very elderly couple.

My patient, Mrs Smith, was on the far side of the bed, and an elderly gentleman, whom I presumed to be her husband, lay on the near side. Also on the bed was a large ginger tomcat that clearly took exception to my presence. Aroused from its slumbers, it rose to its feet, arched its back and glared at me. Its fur bristled, it bared its claws and snarled in an alarming fashion.

'Hello,' I said. 'I'm a specialist from the hospital. Dr Bennett asked me to call.'

There was no response.

I tried again. 'From the hospital,' I repeated, louder this time, assuming that they were both deaf. 'I've come to see you about that lump in your breast.'

There was still no response; it was if I hadn't spoken; just two blank faces staring back at me. Again I tried to explain who I was, and why I was visiting but even after repeating myself a couple of time, they still didn't understand. All the while, I kept a wary eye on the cat, fearful it was about to launch itself at me.

Now, since both husband and wife were obviously extremely deaf, I glanced around looking for any sign of a hearing-aid, but to no avail, so I used sign language to indicate to Mr Smith that I needed to examine his wife. He would have to get up to allow his wife to move to the near side of the bed. Unfortunately, he simply didn't understand what was required, so I assisted him out of the bed, gently but firmly overcoming his objections, and settling him into a chair in the corner. Happily, the cat decided to follow him.

I tried to take a history from Mrs Smith but failed to get an account of her symptoms despite repeated attempts. I began to wish I'd arranged for Dr Bennett to accompany me for this consultation; it would have made things so much easier.

Dr Bennett's message had said that the cancer was obvious, so I presumed that in this particular instance, the patient's story was less important than the examination. I motioned to her to move across to my side of the bed, so I could examine her. She didn't move an inch, so I reached across, slipped my arms under her frail body and attempted to lift her towards me. Her reaction was dramatic. Waving frantically to her husband and squealing like a pig, wriggled like an eel and slipped from my grasp. I tried a second time, unfortunately with the same result. I didn't try a third time, afraid that the neighbours would hear the commotion, rush around and wonder what the hell I was doing.

Having come so far, though, I was determined not to go away without completing my objective, so I jumped up and knelt on the bed where the old man had been lying. It was the first time, and I hope the last, that I would perform a breast examination, kneeling on a bed next to my patient! It was almost impossible for me to keep my balance on the soft mattress. There was an alarming tendency for me to topple forward on top of my patient.

I pulled the bedclothes down to her waist, then reached under the sheets to lift up her nightdress. I heard a movement behind me and turned, anxious to check that the cat was still behaving itself. Fortunately, it was. The noise though came from Mr Smith, who had his hands raised in the air and appeared to be trying to reach me. I smiled at him, assured him I knew what I was doing, and returned to my examination.

Laying my hands on my patient, I performed a detailed examination of both breasts. However, to my surprise, I found no abnormality on either side. I knew Dr Bennett to be a sound practitioner; it was not like him to make an incorrect diagnosis, and he had said the cancer was very obvious. Perplexed, I examined again but merely confirmed that Mrs Smith had two perfectly normal, atrophied, post-menopausal breasts.

Annoyed that I'd made a wasted journey and spoiled my evening, I covered Mrs Smith with the bedclothes, offered a handshake to Mr Smith, which rather rudely, I thought, he declined, and I departed, locking the front door behind me, and replacing the key as I did so.

Later that evening, I rang Dr Bennett and explained that I could find no abnormality in Mrs Smith's breasts at all. I also commented that I felt lucky to have escaped without being attacked by the aggressive cat.

'I don't remember there being any animals when I visited,' he said.

'Yes,' I said, 'I large ginger tomcat which hissed and snarled at me whilst I did the examination.'

'Mrs Smith doesn't have any cats,' he said. 'Where on earth you have been?'

'Number 6, St George's Road.'

There was a long pause.

'Ah, that explains it,' Dr Bennett said. 'My Mrs Smith lives in St George's Street.'

For a few moments, I was totally shell-shocked. What the hell had I done? I'd walked into a stranger's house without a 'by your leave' and sexually assaulted an elderly lady in her own bed. No wonder her husband had looked aggrieved! Then, I confess, the funny side of the matter struck me.

The next day I told the theatre staff what had happened. They thought it was hilarious, and made up a dozen potential headlines for the local paper. Some were quite amusing, others somewhat disturbing.

'Surgeon in sex attack on a local resident.'

'Surgeon struck off the medical register by General Medical Council for sexual assault.'

Thought for the day

When I make a mistake, it's a beaut.

Fiorello H. La Guardia 1882 - 1947

Upsetting our European Friends!

Our first year at Medical School had been tough - in fact, very tough. For three long terms, we had been required to memorise a vast amount of factual information, mainly anatomical detail, which actually proved to be of little relevance when we subsequently qualified as doctors. Frustratingly, we had yet to meet a single patient. I was disillusioned, dispirited, and broke.

Needing a complete change, something to refresh me before resuming my studies after the summer vacation, I decided to take a break, to go abroad, learn a language and earn some money but also, and importantly, to have a good time!

Knowing it would be more fun if I had company, I persuaded my good friend and fellow student, Ben Dyson, to come with me. Together, we applied for posts in a number of European countries but, in the end, settled for positions as 'Practical Nurses' at the Burgerspital, the main hospital in Basel, Switzerland. When signing on we had little idea of what the job entailed, but it proved to be a rewarding experience. Unsurprisingly, we weren't allowed to carry much responsibility, but we learned a lot, generally made ourselves useful and became familiar with ward routine, which incidentally was to make life easier for us when we returned home and were introduced to clinical work.

We spent eight weeks in Basel, and on our last night, we had a party with our new-found Swiss friends to say 'goodbye'. The party proved to be a lively affair, much strong Swiss bier was consumed and a good time was had by all. At the bitter end, in the wee small hours of the morning, Ben and I found ourselves on the roof of the eight-storey building, in our scrubs, looking down at the ambulances in the courtyard below. Quite how we got there, I do not recall, but I confess we were both the worse for wear. Dimly, through bloodshot eyes, we saw two flagpoles, each bearing a flag. One was the Swiss national flag, the other the flag of the canton of Basel. As one does when one is young, irresponsible, and drunk, we pulled the ropes to lower the flags and, by some mischance, finding our scrub trousers in our hands, we tied one pair to the Swiss flag, the other to the Basel flag. We raised both flags again, now with our pants dangling from them, then crept through the corridors in our underwear and went to bed.

Next morning, we were up early to make the journey back to the UK, but before we departed, I took a photo as a souvenir of the two 'flags' flying proudly over the Burgerspital. We then jumped on the tram to the Bahnhof, boarded the train to Calais, and went home.

End of story – or so I thought!

Some thirty-five years later, I was at a Past President's Dinner of the European Gastroenterological Society in Stockholm. There were about twenty of us around the dining table, and after the meal, during the easy conversation that follows when old friends are reunited and have been generously wined and dined, I mentioned what we had done all those years ago, just for fun. There was a sudden exclamation from a Norwegian physician, Jacob Erikssen, a man whom I knew well.

'Johan!! When was this?' he asked.

I did some quick arithmetic in my head.

'Towards the end of August 1972,' I replied.

He stood up suddenly, looking pale and shocked. The room fell silent.

'Oh, my God,' he exclaimed, 'Oh my God, it was you!!! Do you have any idea what happened that day??'

Cheerfully, I said that I hadn't a clue.

He explained that he had undertaken his medical training in Basel and one Friday morning in August 1972, the whole school of 250 or so students had been summoned to the main lecture theatre, and told to sit and wait. At 10 am, the Dean of the Medical School entered, accompanied by the Mayor and the Chief of the Basel Police. The Dean explained that during the night a criminal act, indeed, an act of treason had occurred.

The National Flag of Switzerland and the Basel Cantonal flag of which they were so proud, had been defiled. They had concluded that this could only have been the work of a medical student. Angrily, they stated that whoever had done this dastardly deed would be expelled. If they were a foreign national, they would be deported! They were told they would all remain in the lecture theatre until someone owned up, all day if necessary.

After three hours when no-one had confessed, a process of individual interviews was started. These lasted till 6 pm when, angry and frustrated, the three officials relented and allowed the students to go. They had been allowed no food to eat and only water to drink.

'We were really scared and fed up,' Jacob said. 'It was a terrible day. I remember it clearly. And, oh my God, they were right. It was medical students, but not Swiss students, they were from MANCHESTER!! It was YOU!!'

(Based on a story by Professor Steve Spiro)

Thought for the day

Alcohol ...... enables Parliament to do things at eleven at night that no sane person would do at eleven in the morning.

George Bernard Shaw 1856 - 1950

Sexual Harassment

When Dr Richard Alexander went to work on that lovely spring morning in April 2010, he had no idea he would come within an inch of an accusation of sexual harassment. When I say *'an inch'*, I mean a metaphorical inch, not the sort of *'inch'* of which a blue comedian might speak, when telling a men's locker-room joke, after the nine o'clock watershed! Let me explain.

David Brain was a young, good-looking bachelor who fancied himself with the ladies. His name was entirely appropriate for he was a bright, quick-witted individual; indeed, many thought he should be making more of his life than working for a company that specialised in the demolition of old buildings. Equally, had his name been David Brawn that would have been equally apposite, for he was a tough, muscular individual, who regularly worked out in the gym. He was also a county rugby player and regarded as a possible future international.

Because his job brought him into contact with asbestos, he was required to undergo a statutory annual medical examination. The examination was a requirement of the Health and Safety Executive's control of Asbestos Regulations, as modified to be compliant with the European Commission's Directive (83/477/EEC) relating to individuals exposed to the risks of asbestos at work! This is not the place for me to start a discussion on the merits or otherwise of Brexit - so I won't!

The regulations require a physical examination as well as a lung-function test, so an appointment was made for him to see Dr Alexander, a general practitioner who had a particular interest in industrial medicine.

A couple of weeks before, Dr Alexander, ('Rickie' to his friends and 'Dr Rickie' to many of his patients), had undergone hip replacement surgery. Thankfully, his convalescence was proceeding smoothly; indeed, he was pottering about easily and climbing stairs without any difficulty. For the first few days, he had mobilised using a pair of elbow crutches but, having a positive attitude, he had already discarded one of them.

Further, being a conscientious doctor, eager to return to work, and aware that his absence was placing an extra strain on his partners; he was back in the surgery seeing patients within three weeks of his operation. In truth, this was at a stage of his convalescence, when any of his patients who had undergone a similar procedure, would still be off work. Indeed, he readily acknowledged that had such a patient consulted him, even those employed in a sedentary occupation, he would undoubtedly have given them a sick note.

Dr Rickie had already seen three patients before David Brain arrived. One man had a back injury caused by heavy lifting, another needed his blood-lead level estimating, following occupational exposure while burning through steel girders painted with red lead, and the third patient required an examination for retirement on the grounds of ill health.

When David entered the room, Dr Rickie placed his elbow crutch behind his chair, introduced himself, and then invited the patient to sit. He apologised for being a little immobile but explained about his recent operation. He then embarked on his medical assessment.

He asked David some routine, standard questions, completed the necessary paperwork then, needing to examine his patient's chest, asked him to go behind the screen and undress. He only needed him to strip to the waist, but when David reappeared, he was wearing only a pair of white cotton briefs which emphasised his pleasantly-tanned and well-toned muscular frame. Although Dr Rickie was as straight as a die, he couldn't fail to be impressed!

Dr Rickie rose from his chair, using his elbow crutch to walk around the desk. He then hung the crutch loosely over his arm. Taking his stethoscope out of his pocket, he listened to the back of his patient's chest, without realising that the handpiece of the elbow crutch was swinging gently to and fro against his patient's buttocks.

David became anxious, and his whole body tensed up. He took a step forward.

'Hey, keep still, will you?' Dr Rickie said. He took a stride forward to continue his examination. Inevitably, the crutch, still oscillating gently, followed suit, now creating more pressure than before! David's entire body became rigid. He stopped breathing and slowly turned his head to look over his shoulder.

His facial expression was a mixture of concern and anger. He looked down at his own backside then up at the doctor. He relaxed and laughed.

'F***ing hell, Doc,' he said, 'thank God that's not what I thought it was!'

(Based on a story by Dr R Marcus)

On bisexuality: It immediately doubles your chances of a date on a Saturday night.

Woody Allen

Down to Earth with a Bump

Although the game was only fifteen minutes old, I was enjoying myself as never before. I'd always enjoyed playing football, fancying myself as a winger, but had only ever been an average performer: second team at school, and occasional reserve for the club in the suburb where I lived.

Today though, turning out for the first time with this new team, I was playing the game of my life; I was brilliant! Of course, as the years had slipped by, I'd lost a bit of speed, but I found I could easily outpace the fullback I was up against, even though he looked to be ten or a dozen years younger. Better still, I'd already scored a goal, my first for over a year. I was brim full of confidence. Perhaps my footballing days weren't over after all!?

Suddenly, a loose ball came to me at the edge of the box. I beat my opposite number to it, glided past another defender and slipped the ball past the onrushing goalkeeper as he dived, rather clumsily, I thought, at my feet. Another amazing bit of skill - and another goal! Never mind Ryan Giggs and Georgie Best, here comes a fresh young talent. Well, perhaps not so young, but certainly a new talent. As we walked back to the centre circle to restart the game, my new teammates were full of praise.

'Fine goal! Well done.'

We kicked off again and once more, I dribbled passed the full-back. This time I crossed the ball in the air, but the centre-forward fluffed his header. Nevertheless, I'd created another great scoring opportunity. I was on top of the world, enjoying every moment.

Then disaster! Something happened which burst my bubble, destroyed my confidence, and shattered my ego. Again, I had the ball on the wing. The centre-forward was a big fellow with red hair. He called for me to cross, but his words stopped me in my tracks, they jarred, they were so completely out of place.

'Pass the ball over here please, Mr Sykes, Sir!'

I hesitated and then stopped. The ball was taken off me by the opposition, as the cold reality dawned on me. It was as if I'd been doused by a bucket of cold water. I was now a consultant. They weren't trying to beat me; they were deliberately letting me win! No longer was I a junior doctor able to muck in with the rest; I'd crossed an invisible line. I wasn't one of *'us'*, I was now one of *'them'*.

I should have realised sooner, for there had been other things I'd noticed since taking up my consultant post the previous week. Doors had magically opened for me as I walked along the hospital corridors, the junior doctors took their feet off the chairs, and stood whenever I entered the office, and the nurses offered me tea and biscuits at the end of each ward round. But most disturbing of all - my name had changed. No longer was it *'Hi Peter'*, it was now *'Good Morning, Sir'*, *'How are you today, Sir?'*

Sadly, I realised that I hadn't suddenly and magically acquired phenomenal new sporting skills. My footballing days were over. It was time to hang up my boots and start my new life as a consultant.

Thought for the day

Pride goeth before destruction and a haughty spirit before a fall.

Book of Proverbs

What a Smell

The next patient's problem was apparent to anyone with a sensitive nose, long before the team arrived at his bedside. The smell was that of a putrid decomposing, animal carcase. Powerful and offensive, the odour drifted freely down the ward, undiminished by the deodorant that had been placed on the bedside locker. It was the smell of a badly infected in-growing toenail.

When Mr Rathbone, the Consultant Surgeon and his team reached the patient, the screens were pulled around his bed.

'Sister, can you remove that foul dressing and let us see the nature of this disagreeable problem,' the consultant said, his nose wrinkled in disgust.

Sean, the Surgical Registrar, had seen some unpleasant infections in his time, but few worse than this. The toenail was lost in a sea of pus, and the whole foot was swollen and covered in livid red streaks. The pain caused must have been intense. As the soiled bandages were removed, the smell became almost overpowering.

'Possem secare eius pedes oderem removere,' commented Mr Rathbone grinning at the medical students. *'I could cut off his foot to get rid of the smell'.*

The patient was a tall, gaunt, distinguished-looking man, with white hair and a thin, whispy beard of the same colour. He looked surprised, then angry.

'Aut linguam exideam ut humanitates emendet,' he replied coldly, as he glared at the surgeon, over the top of his half-moon glasses. *'Or cut off his tongue to improve his manners'.*

Mr Rathbone looked startled, then ashamed.

'Look,' he stammered, red-faced, 'I'm most awfully sorry, I never....'

But the patient interrupted him and gave him a lesson, both in good manners and in Latin grammar. 'Actually, Mr Rathbone, you were in error when you used a 'purpose clause' – the purpose of the amputation would be to get rid of the smell. In such a clause, the verb should be in the subjunctive mood. Therefore to be absolutely correct, you should have used 'ut' instead of the infinitive. You should have said *'Possem secare eius pedes ut odorem removerem'."*

'Sir, I apologise most sincerely,' Mr Rathbone began again, 'I wouldn't have spoken in Latin had I any idea....'

Again he was interrupted. 'You wouldn't have spoken in Latin had you known I was the Professor of Classical Studies at the University, but it wouldn't have mattered had I been unable to understand. Is that what you were trying to say?'

Everyone on the ward round, Sean, Sister, and her nursing staff, as well as all the medical students, knew that was exactly what the consultant intended. Yet none of them was particularly upset that Mr Rathbone was getting his 'comeuppance'! Ever since becoming a consultant, Mr Rathbone had criticised and demeaned his students and junior staff. He delighted in embarrassing them in front of their peers or in front of the nurses. Now he was on the receiving end and was clearly not enjoying it. There was a long, uneasy silence.

Finally, Mr Rathbone spoke. 'Sir, I apologise. I should have known better. May I be allowed to start again?'

'You may,' the Professor replied, though his censure of the consultant remained incomplete. 'I have come to seek your advice about this exceedingly painful toe. I know the smell is offensive. I had presumed that as a doctor, you would understand the odour is a symptom of my condition, not a sign of poor personal hygiene. So, yes, it would be best if you started again and perhaps this time we can conduct the consultation in a more civilised fashion.'

Sean had never seen his consultant so visibly shaken. As the round continued, as each bed was reached, he listened in silence as the house officer presented the patient to him, agreed with the management that he suggested, and then moved on without comment.

The round was completed in record time, and Mr Rathbone then departed without a single word or a backward glance. Presumably, he wanted to lick his wounds in private!

'Well, what did you make of that?' Sean asked when the consultant was safely out of earshot.

'Thoroughly deserved,' Sister replied. 'Let's hope it's taught him a lesson.'

Thought for the day

Away with him! Away with him! He speaks Latin.

William Shakespeare 1564 – 1616

Pain and prejudice

Bert Jackson presented to the hospital one evening complaining of abdominal pain at a time when it was my misfortune to be the doctor on duty. He was a Bill Sikes figure: short, muscular, thick-necked, heavily-tattooed, with a mean unsmiling face topped by a crew cut. His dark eyes challenged anyone who dared to meet his gaze, and his chin, covered in grey stubble, was thrust forward aggressively. He would have looked more at home in a dark back alley accompanied by a couple of Rottweiler dogs, each with metal-studded collars, than sitting in a cubicle in Casualty.

My attempts to take his medical history were met with brief, blunt, evasive answers, which were delivered in a loud belligerent voice. His attitude appeared to be 'Look, I've had this pain in my belly for several days now – sort it out.' He didn't see the relevance of the questions I was asking in my attempt to discover the cause of his troubles. He seemed to think I could wave a magic wand, and relieve his pain simply by looking at him and, furthermore, that it was my fault if I couldn't! Eventually, I learned that his pain had been present for four or five days, was worse on the right side than on the left, and was gradually getting worse. These symptoms suggested appendicitis, though they were certainly not typical.

Most patients with an inflamed appendix will be sufficiently tender within 24 hours for the diagnosis to become definite, but when I came to examine Mr Jackson's abdomen, the tenderness was not particularly severe or localised. The next step, and an essential one in the diagnosis of lower abdominal pain, was to perform a rectal examination. However, when I told him of the proposed examination, I was told in a forthright and succinct fashion; 'Forget it Doc, there's no bloody way that you're going to stick your f***ing finger up my f***ing backside!'

His temperature was raised, and his blood tests showed some slight abnormalities, though nothing specific. I thought his troubles were probably due to appendicitis, but was far from certain. It could easily have been gastroenteritis or even diverticulitis. It was clear, however, he needed to be admitted, though probably for observation, rather than for immediate surgery.

When a diagnosis is in doubt, it's a useful exercise to admit the patient for monitoring and observation; this allows the passage of time to clarify the situation. In many cases, symptoms disappear, and the patient regains full health without any diagnosis ever being made. The illness is then ascribed to some self-limiting condition, such as a viral illness. In other cases, time allows the symptoms to become more definite and the diagnosis becomes clear.

I spoke with Mr Khan, my immediate superior, on the phone. He agreed Mr Jackson should be admitted, promising to review him as soon as he was free. I rang the ward, made the necessary arrangements for admission and then, pleased to see the back of an unpleasant man, returned to my Casualty duties.

Shortly after the night staff came on duty, I had a telephone call from the ward.

'I'm sorry to trouble you, Dr Lambert,' Sister said, 'but I have a problem. Mr Jackson won't allow Mr Khan to examine him; he won't even talk to him and he's being extremely rude and aggressive.'

'Why, for heaven's sake?'

'I'm afraid it's because of his colour.'

I went to the ward to resolve the problem, not anticipating any particular difficulty, believing that Mr Jackson's pain, and a natural desire to return to good health would overcome any colour prejudice he might have. He needed to be assessed by an experienced surgeon, and probably required emergency surgery. Without it, he might deteriorate, even die. He needed Mr Khan's expertise and I had little doubt that when the position was explained to him, he would see sense.

When I arrived on the ward, Mr Khan was sitting in the office.

'I'm sorry about this, Paul.' he said, 'It's a long time since this last happened to me.'

'I'm sorry too. I thought this sort of attitude was a thing of the past.'

Mr Khan looked at me rather strangely, but said nothing.

The screens had been pulled around Mr Jackson's bed, and the patients in the vicinity seemed unusually quiet, and looked rather anxious. They were clearly aware of the nature of the problem.

'Is there some sort of difficulty?' I asked.

'Of course there is. I'm not having any f***ing Paki examining me!' Mr Jackson shouted.

'I presume you're talking about Mr Khan.'

'I don't care what his bloody name is.'

'Listen,' I said, 'he's not from Pakistan. His parents were originally from India but he's actually a British citizen, just as you and I are. He holds a British passport.'

'I don't care where he comes from. He could have come from Timbuktu for all I care. He's a wog and he's not laying a finger on me.'

I felt my blood beginning to boil, but tried to keep my voice calm and quiet as I answered.

'He happens to be a very fine surgeon and an extremely capable doctor. For the sake of your own health, you require his expertise right now. He needs to examine you so we can be sure what's causing your pain. In particular, we need to know whether or not you have appendicitis, and whether you require an operation.'

'But you said I did have appendicitis.'

'No, I didn't. I said I thought appendicitis was the most likely diagnosis, but I'm extremely junior, I've not had a lot of experience. I've only been a doctor for a few months. I can't decide whether this is appendicitis or whether you need surgery. And I certainly can't operate on you. Surely you want to be cured?'

'Who's the boss round here?'

'Mr Potts is the consultant.'

'Well, he can bloody well see me instead.'

'Look,' I said trying to be conciliatory, 'there really is no need for that. Mr Khan is a very good doctor and you really ought to let him see you.'

'Look, I've already bloody told you. No Paki doctor is laying a finger on me. Get Potts to see me.'

'I'll see what I can do,' I said in a resigned voice.

Returning to the office, I discussed the situation with Mr Khan. Neither of us wanted to involve the consultant but felt there really was no alternative.

When the switchboard put me through to Mr Potts' home, it was Mr Potts himself who picked up the phone.

'Good evening, Sydney Potts speaking.'

'Good evening, Sir, I'm sorry to trouble you at home in the evening; this is Dr Lambert speaking.'

He sounded surprised. 'Oh, hello Lambert, is everything alright at the hospital? Is there some sort of problem?'

If a case required consultant advice, he would normally expect to be contacted by the registrar, not by his lowly house officer.

'Yes, I'm afraid we have a problem on the ward Sir. I've admitted a man who refuses to be seen by Mr Khan.' I went on to explain the details of the case and the patient's attitude to being examined by Mr Khan.

There was a momentary pause whilst he thought.

'It isn't right that we should be bullied, but equally, I suppose we have a responsibility to stop the patient coming to any harm, even self-inflicted harm.'

There was a further longish pause before Mr Potts spoke again.

'You say, Lambert, that you think this is appendicitis but you're not completely sure.'

'That's right, Sir.'

'Right. Well, I suggest that you leave him on the ward overnight and we'll review him in the morning. If the diagnosis isn't definite, I don't suppose he'll come to any great harm. Oh, and Lambert, don't write him up for any pain relief. That way, by morning, if he really has got appendicitis, we may find that his pain overcomes his prejudice.'

He rang off and I explained the gist of the conversation to Mr Khan. Since the boss had said the patient was to have no analgesia, we would obviously follow his instructions, but I wondered whether it was justifiable, indeed ethical, to leave him in pain. Mr Khan, however, said it was wholly acceptable, indeed, it was good medical practice.

'The more analgesia you give, the more it masks the patient's symptoms, and the more difficult it becomes to make a diagnosis. If you fill the patient with morphine, you take away their pain, and you may be misled into thinking he's getting better.'

I returned to Mr Jackson's bedside and explained what had been agreed with Mr Potts.

Mr Jackson looked triumphant and turned to the patients in the neighbouring beds who were listening to our conversation.

'There you are, I told you so, we don't need any bloody Paki doctors. The whole lot of them should be sent back to 'Paki-land', or whichever damn country they came from.'

It was infuriating to hear such arrogance and prejudice, but he was my patient and it wasn't my place to tackle him on his racist views.

The next day, on our morning ward round, Mr Khan and I found that

Sister had put Mr Jackson into one of the side wards. Apparently the men in neighbouring beds had been so angry at his attitude towards Mr Khan, for whom they had great respect, that a number of them had challenged him. Angry words had been exchanged, the atmosphere on the ward had become difficult and to defuse the situation, the Night Sister had thought it best to segregate Jackson.

As we embarked on the round, Sister suggested it would be wise to see Mr Jackson first.

'He's in a lot of pain now', she said, 'and I suspect he'll end up in theatre having his appendix taken out fairly soon. Oh,' she added to me, with an apologetic glance at Mr Khan, 'I think that you and I had better see him on our own; I'm afraid he's still being extremely stupid and very unpleasant.'

Mr Khan stayed in the office whilst Sister and I entered the side ward and it was immediately apparent that Sister was correct; Mr Jackson was indeed in a great deal of pain. When I examined him, the tenderness in the right lower abdomen was severe, well localised and he now had a significant fever. Despite my inexperience, I was in no doubt that the diagnosis was acute appendicitis. Again, I tried to persuade him to allow Mr Khan to examine him but, despite his severe pain, the patient remained adamant.

'No, if you can't sort it out, get Potts to sort it out.'

Promising to ring the consultant, Sister and I left the room and discussed the situation with Mr Khan.

'I think you'd better ring Mr Potts again, Paul,' he said, 'and see what he has to say. In the meantime, Sister and I will see the rest of the patients.'

For a second time, I rang Mr Potts and gave him an update of the situation.

'You say the patient still won't allow Khan to see him?'

'I'm afraid that's right, Sir.'

'And how definitely do you think that this is appendicitis?'

'Well, I'm fairly certain now, Sir. He's extremely tender in exactly the right spot. He nearly jumps off the bed when you touch him there. I don't think there's a lot of doubt about it.'

'Okay, then arrange the theatre and get on with it.'

I wasn't quite sure what he meant. 'Will you be coming in to perform the operation Sir?'

'No, Khan will do it. Just keep him out of sight until the patient is asleep. Oh – and let's hope the anaesthetist has a white face,' he added.

I returned to Mr Jackson, explained that I'd spoken with Mr Potts, and he had agreed that his appendix should be removed. I said the operation would be performed within the next couple of hours and invited him to sign the standard consent form agreeing to *'removal of appendix and any other procedure that might be required'*. I hoped he wouldn't notice the small print on the bottom of the form which stated that *'no assurance has been given that this operation will be performed by any particular surgeon'*.

Fortunately Mr Jackson did not object to the Caucasian face of the anaesthetist, presumably not realising that he was actually a German national! As the operation got under way, the identification and removal of the appendix proved to be tedious and technically difficult. Partly this was due to the patient's muscular build, but mainly because it was obvious as soon as the abdomen was opened, that the appendix had burst. A large abscess containing pus had formed adjacent to it. Given the five-day history, this was not altogether surprising. The abscess involved adjacent loops of bowel, and these had to be carefully separated before the appendix could be removed. Thanks to Mr Khan's experience, patience, and skill, this was achieved without any damage to these neighbouring structures, though the surgery took over two hours to complete.

As I assisted at the operation, I asked Mr Khan how often he had met such prejudice.

'Only very rarely have I met prejudice as severe as this,' he said, 'but I'm sorry to say that it does exist, indeed, I suppose I'm conscious of it much of the time.'

I expressed surprise, but he went on to explain that there were the obvious things; many white people wouldn't wish their daughter to date or marry a black man, and they would be concerned if such a family moved in next door to them fearing it would reduce the value of their property. But he added that some prejudice was less obvious.

'In the shops or on a bus, the shopkeepers or bus drivers will often be more formal when talking to me or my wife than they would if talking to you. And my children don't seem to get invited to birthday parties quite as often as some of the other children. And in a queue waiting for a bus or a train, if spontaneous conversation springs up between strangers, my family and I tend to be excluded.'

'Well, at least we're free of prejudice within the hospital,' I said.

Mr Khan stopped what he was doing for a moment and looked at me over the top of his surgical mask.

'How I wish that were true,' he said quietly, 'but I have to say that you're wrong, Paul. There's a great deal of prejudice within the National Health Service.'

Again he surprised me. I found this statement difficult to believe.

'But surely nobody is prejudiced against you,' I said. 'The nurses, doctors and consultants here all greatly value your contribution. This team would fall apart if you weren't here to keep it going. And if I ever needed an operation I should be very happy for you to perform it for me. This is the only patient who hasn't been grateful to you for your care and attention. All the other patients greatly appreciate your help, and last night they expressed that view openly. That's why this man has ended up in a side ward.'

'Oh, I know I'm appreciated here, and I know I do good work,' Mr Khan said, 'but you're wrong if you think there's no prejudice. I've been a registrar for a long time now. I'm a fellow of the Royal College of Surgeons, I've written a couple of research papers and have a stronger CV than any of the other registrars in the hospital, but I miss out when I apply for a more senior post. Most registrars get promoted after three or four years, I've already been here for seven years. I've got better qualifications and more experience, but junior people leapfrog over me. Actually, I suspect it suits Mr Potts to keep me here as his registrar. With my experience, there are very few emergencies which I can't manage without his support. It means he rarely has to come into the hospital to deal with out-of-hours problems.'

He was speaking quietly, and didn't appear angry, indeed it sounded as if he accepted the situation philosophically.

He continued, 'And consider the wider picture. You've only got to look where most overseas doctors work. We have a few here in the teaching hospital but the vast majority work in district general hospitals, where the job prospects are less good. As you know, it's almost impossible to be appointed as an NHS consultant unless you do the majority of your training in a teaching hospital, so overseas doctors working in the periphery have even less chance of promotion than I do.'

I hadn't considered this before but had to admit that he was correct. I knew that in some hospitals nearly all the junior hospital doctors were overseas trainees. Then he asked a question that really made me think.

'Why is it that people always refer to me as Mr Khan and yet they refer to the other registrars and to you by your Christian name?'

On reflection, I had to acknowledge this was true. The sisters on the ward invariably used the prefix 'Mister' when referring to Mr Khan and indeed so did I. Was that because I felt it was a complement; a mark of respect to indicate that I regarded him as a good surgeon or was I displaying a degree of prejudice, albeit subconsciously? I had never thought I was in the least prejudiced but could it be that at some deeper level, I did regard him as being 'different'?

He continued in lighter mood, 'Mind you, colour prejudice isn't the only prejudice within the health service. What about the prejudice against women? How many female consultants do you know? Do you know any female consultant surgeons?'

The truth was that I didn't. I knew of several female radiologists and one or two anaesthetists; specialties in which the competition for consultant posts was a little less fierce, but surgery was entirely a male preserve.

Mr Khan glanced at the staff nurse who was acting as scrub nurse for this particular operation.

'Mind you; perhaps it's as well there are no female surgeons,' he said provocatively, 'I'm not sure that the female personality is suited to the rigors of a career in surgery. Women aren't as tough as men, are they, and wouldn't be able to stand the long hours and the exacting work?'

He had cleverly changed the focus of the conversation and it was obvious to me he was only teasing, but the Staff Nurse didn't see it that way and was quick to respond.

'You're just as prejudiced as he is,' she said, indicating the patient, 'women are every bit as good as men, if not better, and they would make wonderful surgeons. Furthermore, if we did have some female surgeons, they wouldn't walk around with the fancy airs and graces that some of the consultants in this hospital have.'

I looked across the table at Mr Khan, and for a moment neither of us spoke. It was clear we both thought it wiser not to ask her to give examples.

'You're quite right, Staff Nurse,' said Mr Khan, who had decided to pour oil on troubled waters. 'I'm sure women have manual dexterity equal, if not superior to that of men and, by and large, they are much more patient, both of which traits would make them good technical operators in theatre. Generally, their communication skills are better too. But they will continue to be disadvantaged whilst it takes 10 to12 years to train, especially as much of that time is spent 'on call'. That would require women to make big sacrifices since it's very difficult to train part-time.'

Thereafter, the operation continued in a more light-hearted mood but the procedure had taken more than twice as long as normal, and because of the difficulties encountered on the way, there was a potential for complications in the post-operative period. There had been pus and gross infection around the ruptured appendix, and a wound infection or worse, an infection deep within the abdomen, were distinct possibilities that might lead to a stormy convalescence and a prolonged stay in hospital.

Mr Potts was absent from the Monday morning ward round, so it was only on the fifth post-operative day that he saw Mr Jackson for the first time. As it happened, his recovery had been slow but uneventful, complications having been avoided. When Mr Potts, accompanied by his team of doctors and nurses entered Mr Jackson's side room, I wondered whether he would object to the presence of Mr Khan at his bedside, but possibly because the consultant was present, he said nothing. As usual, in my role as house officer, I presented an abstract of Mr Jackson's treatment to Mr Potts. I made no reference to the problems we had encountered with the patient's prejudice, and certainly didn't mention it was Mr Khan who had performed the procedure, but I did stress, in a voice loud enough for the patient to hear, that the surgery had been technically exacting, had been carried out with a great deal of skill, as a result of which all complications had been avoided.

Mr Potts asked to see the patient's notes. There was a long pause as he turned to the page containing details of the operation which he read carefully before addressing the patient, reinforcing the point I had been making.

'This was a very advanced case of appendicitis, your appendix had ruptured, and there was a very severe infection inside your belly. It was a life-threatening situation. It's as well you had an operation, for without it you might not be here to tell the tale. You have reason to be extremely grateful to the surgeon, and his skill.'

It is strange but true, that patients almost always assume that their consultant performs all the operations on every patient under his care. I have even met patients in the outpatient clinic, attending for their post-surgical review, who believe implicitly that the consultant performed their operation, even though they didn't see him once during the time they were on the ward. In this case, Mr Jackson certainly came to this conclusion and begrudgingly offered his thanks to Mr Potts for looking after him. This was probably the opening the consultant had been engineering.

'You don't need to thank me; you need to thank the surgeon whose skill has saved your life.'

Mr Jackson turned towards me; for once he seemed to be on his best behaviour.

'Thank you, Doc.' he said quietly.

It was Mr Potts who spoke next.

'No. It wasn't Dr Lambert who did your operation; it was Mr Khan, and he is the man you need to thank. He applied his considerable skill and experience to your problem, despite your appalling rudeness to him.

Mr Jackson looked dumbfounded. For quite some time there was silence in the room, until finally he found his voice.

'Ta, doctor,' he managed to mutter, though the words were directed not to Mr Khan but to the floor.

Mr Potts turned to Sister, anger evident in his tone. 'Get this man out of this side ward. There's absolutely no medical reason for him to be here. Side wards are for patients who are seriously ill, not for those who are ignorant and prejudiced.'

He glared at Mr Jackson, then turned and left. With his back to the patient, he didn't see the **V** sign that Mr Jackson gave him as he exited the room.

The patient's wife

Mrs Fielding, Ken's wife, found herself sitting, frightened and alone, in the anaesthetic room. She had accompanied her husband as he was rushed through the hospital corridors from the Emergency Department to the operating theatre. She had sat on a stool and held his hand whilst cannulae were inserted into his arms, and blood pumped into his body. She had whispered words of love and reassurance as the anaesthetic was administered, but when the action had moved into the operating theatre itself, she had been left behind, alone and forgotten. She had his jacket and trousers over her arm, his glasses, wallet, and keys in one hand and a tear-stained handkerchief in the other.

There was a small porthole in the door between the anaesthetic room and the theatre, but she dared not go and see what was happening. Had she done so, she would have been horrified to see the speed with which a huge incision had been made in her husband's abdomen. A religious woman, she recognised how sick he was; she had never seen anyone quite so ill. And he had been as right as rain when he had kissed her goodbye and gone to work that morning. How fragile, how unpredictable was life. She prayed that he would survive.

She had seen the urgency with which he had been treated, and had heeded the surgeon's words when he had been so pessimistic about the chances of a successful outcome. The largest blood vessel in the body has ruptured, he had said, a very grave situation. Now, all she could do was to put her faith in God and her trust in the doctors and nurses. She had been surprised how young the surgeon had looked, yet impressed how calm he seemed, and how efficiently he had arranged for the operation to be performed. She thought how wonderful it was that someone of such tender years should have the experience and expertise to perform surgery for such serious conditions.

She was still there five minutes later when the theatre technician slipped into the room to fetch another bottle of plasma. He was surprised to see her.

'I'm afraid you can't stay here,' he said, wondering where he should advise her to go. 'Do you want to go home, or would you prefer to wait in the hospital?'

'I couldn't possibly go home. I'd like to wait if I may?'

'Normally, you would wait in the ward, but I'm afraid there hasn't been time for your husband to be allocated a bed. Why not wait in the hospital canteen? You can get a drink there, and we can contact you if necessary.'

'How long will it be, do you think?'

'I'm afraid that's impossible to say,' the technician replied gently. He knew that it might be less than ten minutes if the bleeding couldn't be stopped, anything up to three or four hours if the patient survived.

Before she went to the canteen, Mrs Fielding rang her daughter. Thanks to an earlier call, she already knew that her dad had been rushed to the hospital. She had collected her little girl from the nursery and was giving her tea when the call came through. She promised to come as soon as she was able to arrange childcare and get a taxi. Mrs Fielding then went to the canteen, ordered a drink and a biscuit, then, fearing the worst, settled down to wait in a quiet corner.

One hour passed, then a second. Her daughter arrived, and still, she waited, desperate for news. Was the fact that the operation was taking so long a good sign or a bad one, she wondered? Or had her husband already died, and they were afraid to come and tell her?

Every time someone entered the canteen, or the telephone rang, her heart jumped, thinking there might be a message for her. Another thirty minutes passed, and still, no one had contacted her. On and on, she waited.

'I can't bear this any longer,' her daughter finally said. 'Surely, there should be some news by now.'

'You don't think they've forgotten about us, do you? They were so busy with your dad, and it's quite possible.'

'But who can we ask? None of the people in here will know anything about it.'

'I'm going to ask one of the nurses over there. I'm sure they'll know what we should do.'

Hesitantly, she approached a group of nurses who were sitting chatting at a nearby table. One of them went to the canteen phone and rang the theatre on her behalf. She returned a couple of minutes later.

'Your husband's still in theatre,' she said gently. 'I'm afraid you'll just have to wait. But they do know you're here, and they've promised to send someone down to speak with you when they've finished.'

As they waited, Mrs Fielding thought of their time together, their courtship, that embarrassing moment when Ken had been so old-fashioned and formally asked for her hand in marriage, those early days when life had been such a struggle with young children and so little money. And then more recent times, happier times, when their first grandchild was born. What a little joy she was and how Ken loved to play with her. Her arrival had been a godsend when Ken had been so low, having lost his job.

The canteen door opened again, and once more, her heart jumped, but it was only another group of nurses who sauntered to the counter oblivious of the anxiety their entry had caused.

Still, they waited. Apart from a few nurses, they were now the only ones in the room. Mrs Fielding looked at her watch; it was two in the morning, they had been sitting there for nearly four hours. The longer they waited, the more pessimistic she became. Her daughter tried to be optimistic.

'If they're still operating on Dad, he must still be alive; there must be a chance.'

But as the minutes dragged on, her mother began to fear the worst.

'I'm not sure how I'll manage without him,' she said. 'He was such a lovely man, so kind, so thoughtful. I know he got a bit depressed when he was made redundant, but he was the strong one you know, the one who kept us going when things got tough. Do you remember the time when....'

She stopped as once again, the canteen door opened. This time it was the surgeon.

She saw him stop as his eyes scanned the room, looking for them. Then he walked slowly, reluctantly, towards them, his shoulders drooped, his face severe, sadness mixed with the exhaustion in his eyes. She knew exactly what he was going to say before he had even reached them and started to speak.

Peter continues to publish new stories on his blog at www.medicaltales.org where you can Sign On/Subscribe and receive all future tales, free of charge, direct to your email in-box.

.

Lightning Source UK Ltd.
Milton Keynes UK
UKHW041445240420
362136UK00005B/306